BURDENED
AGENCY

BURDENED AGENCY

Christian Theology and End-of-Life Ethics

TRAVIS PICKELL

University of Notre Dame Press
Notre Dame, Indiana

Copyright © 2024 by University of Notre Dame
Notre Dame, Indiana 46556
www.undpress.nd.edu

All Rights Reserved

Manufactured in the United States of America

Library of Congress Control Number: 2024937294

ISBN: 978-0-268-20841-7 (Hardback)
ISBN: 978-0-268-20840-0 (WebPDF)
ISBN: 978-0-268-20896-7 (Epub3)

To

SARAH

This love of ours is no light thing

Give up your self, and you will find your real self. Lose your life and you will save it. Submit to death, death of your ambitions and favourite wishes every day and death of your whole body in the end: submit with every fibre of your being, and you will find eternal life. Keep back nothing. Nothing that you have not given away will ever be really yours. Nothing in you that has not died will ever be raised from the dead.

—C.S. Lewis, *Mere Christianity*

God goes belonging to every riven thing he's made.

—Christian Wiman

Contents

	Acknowledgments	ix
	Introduction: The Landscape of Modern Dying	xi
ONE	Burdened Agency	1
TWO	Scripts for Dying	21
THREE	Persons, Freedom, and a Catholic Spirituality of Martyrdom	39
FOUR	Karl Barth on Agency in Dying: Accepting Creaturely Finitude	61
FIVE	Stanley Hauerwas on Agency in Dying: Ethics of Dispossession	87
SIX	Prayer, Baptism, and Eucharist	113
	Conclusion: Humanity *Sub Specie Mortis*	131
	Notes	151
	Bibliography	181
	Index	201

Acknowledgments

I may never have developed the ideas in this book if my *Doktorvater*, Chuck Mathewes, had not advised me to "start with the end in mind." I certainly would not have finished it without his invaluable mentorship and steadfast encouragement. Nor would it have been quite so fun without his timely sense of humor, penchant for bringing people together to build a sense of academic and intellectual community, or his legendary command of the lunch menu at Peter Chang's. I owe much to Jim Childress, who has been a source of support and a model of what it means to treat every individual with respect and kindness. Margaret Mohrmann, Paul Jones, and James Davison Hunter each read and contributed to this project in its early days. I am grateful for their wisdom and their attention, which have saved me from innumerable mistakes and embarrassments.

I have been blessed to experience several rich environments for academic life and community. This book spans my time at the University of Virginia (UVA), Anselm House, and George Fox University. I am deeply thankful for the intellectual engagement I have experienced in various communities, including the Institute for Advanced Studies in Culture, the Institute for Practical Ethics and Public Life at UVA, the Theology, Medicine and Culture Program at Duke University, the Paul Ramsey Institute, and the Conference on Medicine and Religion.

Over the years, I have had the opportunity to share ideas contained in this book with many colleagues. I thank the following people for being thoughtful friends, collaborators, and mentors along the way: Matthew Puffer, Philip Lorish, John Yoon, Farr Curlin, Brewer Eberly, Wilson Ricketts,

Ashley Moyse, Sumner Abraham, Joseph Clair, Abigail Favale, Patrick Smith, Rick Campanelli, Michael Lamb, and, of course, the Portland Portobellos—Brett McCarty, Ryan Antiel, Tyler Tate, and Brendan Johnson. I want to extend my deepest thanks to Scott and Meg for allowing me to tell part of your story in this book. You all inspire me.

Thanks to Emily King, my editor at the University of Notre Dame Press, for guiding this book through the publication process. Your editorial assistance has improved the book significantly. The faults that remain are my own.

Thank you, Paul and Nancy Lee Gauche, for believing in me and for your constant prayers. Also, thank you for showing me what it looks like to love someone well at the end of their life. I will never forget the dignity and grace with which you treated Eugene and how you refused to allow his final years to be spent alone. And Soren, thanks for being my first and best brother. My parents, Julie and Ray Pickell, and grandparents Kate and Larry Norman always saw the best in me and never let me believe for a minute that I could not accomplish something that I set out to achieve. Because they believed in me, I learned to believe in myself.

One of my advisers told me early on that I should be careful about writing a book about death. "They rarely get finished," she said. Despite the ominous note of the warning, I understand now what she means. I am sure that this topic would have weighed me down were it not for the daily uplifting and joyous presence of my daughters, Ruby, Ryann, and Emily. Thank you for reminding me every day why life is a wonderful gift, full of potential and surprise, if we only have eyes to see. Finally, I dedicate this book to Sarah, sine qua non. "If it's half as good as the half we've known, here's Hail! To the rest of the road" (Van Auken).

Introduction

The Landscape of Modern Dying

In life, there are certain experiences that are both common to all and intensely personal: the experience of childhood and adolescence, the discovery and negotiation of friendships and romantic love, relationships of caring and being cared for, the experience of beauty, the pursuit of truth and justice. Many of these experiences are marked in different religious traditions by rituals of various sorts; all are a perennial source of philosophical and theological thinking. It is the convergence of the quotidian and the singular, the universal and the utterly particular, that explains why these experiences are central sites of religious practice and moral reflection. Death is, of course, one of these experiences.

As Martin Heidegger famously noted, the human being is unique among creatures in recognizing that she is always already "thrown" toward death. One question that occupied his attention was, what will she do with this knowledge? What difference will it make in her life? The relationship she adopts toward her mortal existence is her "ownmost possibility," a question that only she can answer. Heidegger's own suggestion—that a radical transformation toward an authentic existence occurs only through freely adopting a stance of actively "running up" to the death that awaits you— is one potential answer to this question. There are many others. What Heidegger makes clear, however, is that every person adopts a particular *stance* or *attitude* toward death. Now, attitudes can and do change throughout one's life. And attitudes about death and dying often remain subterranean and pre-reflective, lying beneath the surface of one's active attention. But the point is that whether we acknowledge it or not, our posture toward death affects not only how we die but also *the way we live our lives*. Even the apparent failure to adopt a stance toward death itself constitutes a stance toward death. Denial is a posture, too.

Indeed, were it not for an unexpected cancer diagnosis during my first week of graduate school, I would in all likelihood have remained oblivious to my own subconscious stance of death denial. As it happened, I was also tasked that semester with serving as a teaching assistant for a large class on religion and biomedical ethics. Friday afternoons were particularly eventful, as I would lead discussion sections for three hours, then walk down the block to the Emily Couric Cancer Center to receive a regimen of chemotherapy before returning home to recover over the weekend. I do not bring this up to claim any special epistemic authority (although there is something about the process of losing your hair over the course of a semester that makes students pay particular attention when an instructor speaks about end-of-life issues). Rather, I mention it to place myself within the ranks of those who discover the importance of underlying attitudes toward mortality only through an experience of illness and bodily vulnerability.

Our own society does not deal very well with death and dying. Some suggest that this is the result of a widespread cultural attitude of denial. Arthur C. McGill, for example, characterized contemporary America as a nation of *bronze people*, who "live according to an ethic of success or avoidance . . . , [devoting] themselves to expunging from their lives every appearance, every intimation of death."[1] In advertising and popular culture, this ethic of success is reflected in portrayals of old age and retirement that resemble a second adolescence, a period apparently free of bonds of responsibility in which leisure is pursued with carefree abandon and romance blossoms in ways that are impossible in the midst of work and family life. I do not want to suggest that freedom, leisure, and romance are not desirable features at any stage of life—I hope to have my fair share of each even into old age! Nevertheless, the one-sided portrayal of this ideal betrays a cultural discomfort with the ambiguous realities of aging (the loss of mental acuity, for example, or the gaining of folds in the skin) and the eventual fact of death, which these portend.

There are, however, plausible reasons to question the notion that the American attitude toward death is primarily denial. The cultural landscape is complicated. In fact, there seems to be a resurgence of attention to death and dying in the popular media. A couple of generations ago, the "death awareness movement" brought death and dying into the light, largely fueled by a shared recognition that the combination of death's medicalization and its erasure from public consciousness was resulting in an undesirable state of affairs. The type of death that was growing increasingly likely—a death marked by loneliness, social isolation, and overuse of technology—was widely recognized as a "bad" death. In the past few decades, much has changed, but much has also remained the same. Today, major motion pictures and *New York Times* best-selling books and memoirs are increasingly focusing on the end of life, and there seems to be a steady proliferation of newspaper and journal articles exploring the ethical ambiguities of death and dying. Self-proclaimed "transhumanists" have initiated a (still-nascent) public debate about whether, if we were able to do so, it would be desirable to cure the "disease" of old age, ushering in an era of radical life extension. In some cities, "death cafés" are now commonplace. At these public dinners, participants gather to consider their mortality and share their fears and desires for the end of life. It seems like death is finally getting its due. As with the original "death awareness movement," however, this widespread attention reveals a general dissatisfaction with the institutions, practices, and cultural influences surrounding death and dying in our society. A book like Atul Gawande's *Being Mortal* is likely only a wild success in a culture that struggles with being mortal.[2]

Perhaps the most confounding aspect of dying today is the fact that it increasingly must be *chosen*. Death used to be generally understood as something that *happens to* us. In previous eras, a chosen death was an exception to the rule. The soldier throwing himself on a grenade to save his comrades or the dramatic suicides of Shakespeare's *Romeo and Juliet* inspire and move us in their tragic or heroic rarity. But when the dying process is enveloped by the ever-increasing power and dominion of medicine, the exception becomes the rule: today, we are more likely than ever to choose the manner and timing of our deaths (or the death of a loved one). In the illustrious words of Sir Winston Churchill (or was it Spiderman?), with great power comes great responsibility. It is far from clear, however, that such responsibility is welcomed by the average person.

The key concept in this book is a phenomenon I call burdened agency. Briefly put, burdened agency denotes two things simultaneously: (1) the burden of *having-to-choose* means we are increasingly expected to make concrete choices about the manner and timing of death; (2) the burden of *reflexivity* means that we must do so in an increasingly individualistic context with less cultural and religious guidance than ever before. The burden *of* agency combined with the reflexive burden *on* agency often results in an existential predicament of anxiety, bewilderment, and regret. The experience of burdened agency has a way of exposing unreflective posture toward death and dying (both individually and culturally). The process of bringing to light—of making explicit—those subterranean beliefs and attitudes about death and dying is a central task of this book.

Two important caveats suggest themselves at this point. The first has to do with issues of race, class, and gender. I am aware that the account given in this book is one that makes sense most especially from a given social location. I am a well-educated, middle-class, white male, and although I have experienced the role of patient firsthand, my own experience with the medical establishment was shaped by my relatively privileged position. I have never struggled to pay a hospital bill, nor have I gone without health insurance for very long. I also felt no reason to distrust the physicians and nurses who took care of me over the years.

Questions of inequity in access to health care and legacies of institutional racism and sexism are important, though they are not explored in depth in this book. As I will explain in chapter 1, the central issue of burdened agency in not unique to a particular social class, race, or gender, though it will be distinctively filtered through these elements of identity and social location. The problems raised by poverty, sexism, and institutional racism do not so much relieve people of burdened agency, in the sense that I will explain it, but rather constitute *additional* burdens on one's agency. It is my hope that this book will provoke further discussion about exactly these issues.

The second caveat is this: there is a very real danger, given that this book combines a critique of modernity with an ethical analysis of medical practices, that a reader might assume that it represents an "anti-medicine" or "anti–modern medicine" stance. Such an assumption would be misguided. I have every reason to be thankful for modern medicine (the cancer I was diagnosed with would have killed me thirty years ago), and I greatly respect the work of physicians and nurses (I am married to one). This book should be read not as anti-medicine but rather as a sympathetic attempt to enrich the moral and theological discourse about medicine and to encourage, as one author puts it, "the finest traditions of [the] calling."[3]

This book is about the challenges we face in dying well and specifically about how best to understand and bear the responsibilities of choice at the end of life. It is not, however, a guidebook for helping patients and caretakers to navigate the terrain of modern medicine and end-of-life decisions. Rather, it is a study of the contribution of Christian theology for contemporary debates about end-of-life ethics. A few words about this approach are in order, for it will hardly be obvious to some readers what contribution we might expect from religious or theological sources in dealing with a practical problem like burdened agency.

One presupposition of this book is that social norms and institutions are never value-neutral or merely pragmatic arrangements. On the contrary, these norms and institutions reflect and carry forward substantive (if latent or inarticulate) assumptions and beliefs about the nature of the world, humanity, social and political relations, and the moral life. Many of the beliefs that underlie our current end-of-life practices are secularized variants of ideas that originally had their provenance in theological discourse. On some level, all such beliefs are theological or religious in character.[4] Once this connection has been made explicit, such ideals are open to theological analysis and critique (importantly, in this process, theology is also open to critique and revision).

The connections between social practices and the ideals and beliefs embedded in them are not always easy to tease out. It requires, at minimum, attention to the work of social scientists and others who give thick accounts of such institutions and practices as they currently exist and as they have developed over time. Therefore, this book draws heavily on the disciplines of sociology, intellectual history, medical anthropology, history of medicine, and clinical biomedical ethics to describe the conditions under which dying occurs today and to explain how we got here. I then turn to the work of intellectual historians to explicate the substantive beliefs and ideals that are embedded in the social practices of dying that are most common today.

What begins as an inquiry into modern practices and ideals about death and dying opens up into a broader discussion about what it means to be a human being and a moral agent. In light of this, a central theme emerges: we can learn much about a culture's assumptions about moral agency and theological anthropology by attending to that culture's practices of dying and the ethical discourse that surrounds such practices. Correlatively, alternative notions of moral agency and theological anthropology—in this case, Christian theological notions—offer critical leverage for envisioning alternative practices and for better understanding shortcomings of current institutions and norms. Although the issues taken up in this book are relevant to persons of all different religious affiliations (or no affiliation at all), the scope of the theological analysis is limited to Christianity. Even though this book necessarily offers a particular and limited perspective, I believe and hope that it will find sympathetic readers who identify with other religious traditions or who belong to that ever-growing contingent of religious "nones."

There are three audiences to whom this book will likely be of interest. First, for scholars of religion, this study offers (a) an account of the interrelation between religious institutions and practices, on the one hand, and the development and shape of medicine and medical practice, on the other; (b) an analysis of the relationship between religious practice and cultural formation that will be relevant for those interested in broader issues of religion and society; and (c) an explication of specifically Christian religious practices in terms of their relationship with death and dying, on the one hand, and normative vision of moral agency and ethics, on the other. Second, theologians and Christian ethicists will be interested in the account of Christian understandings of death and human agency in dying, especially insofar as these reflect substantive contributions to theological anthropology, as well as to the question of the relationship between the doctrine of creation and the problem of evil. Finally, this book aims to be of some help to academically interested practitioners of medicine (including nurses and other caretakers) as well as any reader who has felt or will likely feel the existential weight of burdened agency. For such readers, the very act of examining these issues will likely provoke moments of self-reflection that are crucial to a healthy engagement with or practice of medicine at the end of life.

The first chapter of this book introduces the concept of burdened agency as an ethical phenomenon. In doing so, it highlights central changes that have occurred with respect to common experiences of dying in modern, Western, industrialized societies. It describes how individuals (patients, proxies, and health-care professionals) are increasingly expected to make decisions about the nature and timing of death. It then explains the concept of "deinstitutionalization" and its effects on moral agency: when social and cultural norms fail to provide guidance to the dying, individuals are forced to seek meaning in a more private, individualistic, and reflexive way. But the conditions of our modern dying—including the social isolation of the elderly and dying, social taboos about discussing death, the changing disease burden and illness trajectories, societal assumptions regarding human suffering and the use of technology, and other institutional realities—generally serve as hindrances to such meaning making and leave individuals in a precarious existential position as they seek to navigate the agency they so ambivalently possess.

Chapter 2 shifts the focus to the moral ontology and philosophical anthropology that underlie both the highly medical dying characteristic of the intensive care unit (ICU) and the two most visible cultural "scripts" for dying that have arisen in response to the ICU—namely, hospice and physician-assisted suicide (PAS). Drawing on Charles Taylor's account of modern identity and modern social imaginaries, I argue that each of these scripts is deeply indebted to the various facets of the modern social imaginary: (a) a sense of inwardness, which locates freedom in the individual will and which locates dignity in the exercise of rational autonomy; (b) the sense that nature constitutes a moral source so that authenticity is located in attunement to nature (conceived in highly individualistic terms), and dignity is understood in terms of self-expression; and (c) the affirmation of ordinary life, including especially the realm of labor and work, on the one hand, and marriage and family life, on the other. During the Enlightenment, the moral ideals of universal benevolence and the affirmation of ordinary life converged to create a moral imperative to reduce suffering and prevent death. Although the relationship between Christianity and this modern social imaginary is complicated, the theological claims and religious practices of Christianity constitute a distinctive standpoint that challenges many of the features just named.

Chapter 3 explicates the teachings about death and dying as they are developed in Roman Catholic moral theology. Beginning with a review of the *Catechism of the Catholic Church*, it then turns to two prominent post–Vatican II accounts of agency in dying. Richard McCormick, S.J., gives a personalist natural-law approach that highlights the relationship between decision making at the end of life and the various goods of a human life considered as a whole. Karl Rahner, S.J., offers a Christian existentialist understanding of death as a personal act and opportunity to demonstrate faithful surrender before the divine. A Catholic approach to agency in dying, I argue, is best summed up in Servais Pinckaers, O.P.'s, notion of a "spirituality of martyrdom," which understands agency in dying as neither "active control" nor "mere passivity" but as "submissive receptivity" of what comes from God's hand for the sake of love. Just as the martyr witnesses to her trust in God's providence by being faithful *unto* death, so also more quotidian and mundane instances of dying can witness to God's lordship when they are approached in the posture of submissive receptivity.

Chapter 4 turns at length to the theology of Karl Barth, which represents a fundamentally different approach to death and human mortality. I trace Barth's understanding of death and dying from his early period (*Der Romerbrief*) to his mature theological reflection of *Church Dogmatics* III.4. I argue, on the one hand, that Barth's treatment of death as an aspect of creaturely existence and his robust theological affirmation of human temporality and finitude provide conceptual resources for understanding death as a natural end, which can be accepted and affirmed as such. On the other hand, however, Barth's dialectical insistence on the association of death with guilt for the human sinner means that death can only be accepted as natural once it is affirmed as also wholly *unnatural*—as that which has been overcome and rejected in Jesus Christ. Seen in this dialectical richness, death becomes a necessary precondition for God's granting of the surplus gift of resurrection *life*. Similar to the spirituality of martyrdom, Barth advocates a posture of receptiveness to human mortality but one that is informed by a concrete appreciation for the gift of human limitedness and boundaries (i.e., creaturely finitude).

Chapter 5 turns to the work of contemporary theologian and social ethicist Stanley Hauerwas. Hauerwas's work represents a synthetic convergence of the Roman Catholic spirituality of martyrdom and the Barthian acceptance of creaturely finitude. I show how these themes inform both his theological method (e.g., the use of the essay form rather than the theological treatise and the emphasis on moral description rather than discrete decision) as well as his ethical convictions (e.g., his refusal of the liberal association between rational agency and human dignity, his eschewal of the presumption that all suffering should be avoided, and his insistence on the value of persons with disabilities). I argue that Hauerwas provides a theological account of an "ethic of dispossession," which finds its original application in a theology of nonviolence but also has particular relevance for understanding the relationship between agency and the experience of advanced aging and, ultimately, death and dying.

In chapter 6, I consider how concrete practices—in both ecclesial and health-care settings—carry forward and sustain these core moral dispositions in ways that challenge the dominant social imaginary. I argue that Christian theologians, ethicists, clergy, and medical practitioners should collaborate in a process of re-embedding the practices of medicine and end-of-life care in the ecclesial narratives and practices so that ordinary people might learn to see and speak of their everyday experience in terms that resist moral logics that lead to the ICU or to an *uncritical* acceptance of the dominant scripts of hospice and euthanasia. The chapter lifts up three Christian practices, noting their implications for clinical practice and Christian dying. Prayer, I argue, is a practice of unselfing, which is ordered toward experiencing an empowering dependence on God. Under this understanding, prayer (and specifically silent prayer or contemplation) enacts a form of agency that runs counter to the modern social imaginary. Baptism seals one's identity in the death and resurrection of Jesus Christ so that in one sense, the Christian's death is always behind her. Baptism prefigures and presages martyrdom, as faithfully dying in the Lord. Finally, in the Eucharist, the Christian is drawn further and further into this identity as she is mysteriously drawn into the broken body of Christ. Approaching the altar with empty hands, Eucharist is also a regular enactment and recognition of one's creaturely dependence and eccentric existence. These elements make Eucharist an act of Christian *kenosis*, or self-emptying—a displacement of the self that makes room for God. Each of these practices inculcates an alternative form of agency, thereby subverting the drive toward mastery and control at the heart of medical culture and modern society. Individuals may not be able to fully avoid burdened agency, but this shift, I argue and will endeavor to demonstrate, can help them bear the burden more faithfully and humanely.

ONE

Burdened Agency

DEATH: THE UNCERTAIN CERTAINTY?

Søren Kierkegaard, with characteristic paradox, urged his readers to remember that death is, at one and the same time, "the only certainty and the only thing about which nothing is certain."[1] *That* death will come to each and every person is beyond doubt; *when* and *how* it will occur is unknowable. Death may come at any moment ("*Then*, all is over!") because it lies outside of human control. *Mors certa, hora incerta.*

There is something intuitively right about this. For the majority of people, when death arrives, it does so with some element of surprise, even if preceded by a long period of decline. While a cloaked figure with a scythe may not actually knock at our door, we have a sense that death *comes* to us—we know not when. At the same time, the *uncertainty* of death (in this Kierkegaardian sense) may be eroding in the developed West.

Consider the following two cases. The first case involves Mrs. Faith Carver, ninety-two, who lives in a nursing home in Fresno, California. She is a longtime widow with no family nearby. Because she suffers from advanced dementia, she does not recognize friends and family, and she relies on the help of nursing staff to complete even the simplest tasks, like bathing, dressing, and eating. One morning, she develops a high fever and is transferred to a local emergency room for treatment. There, she is diagnosed with pneumonia. Because her chart contains no living will or advance directive indicating her preferences for care, the physician contacts her family, who are "understandably reluctant to withhold life-prolonging treatments." Mrs. Carver is transferred to the intensive care unit (ICU), where she receives intravenous antibiotics and is intubated to provide her with sustenance, for she can no longer take foods orally. Soon after being placed in the ICU, she goes into cardiac arrest. "An emergency code [is] called over the loudspeaker and a team [is] summoned to perform CPR [cardiopulmonary resuscitation], invading the body with tubes, compressing the chest hard enough to pump blood manually . . . and applying electrical jolts to try shocking [her] heart back into a rhythm." Eventually, the attending physician declares these efforts futile, and Faith Carver is allowed to die.[2]

The second case involves Dr. Richard Wesley, sixty-seven. Dr. Wesley's mind is sharp and lucid. He can banter with his family and is constantly cracking jokes. His body, however, is deteriorating rapidly. Dr. Wesley has amyotrophic lateral sclerosis (ALS), also known as Lou Gehrig's disease. ALS is an incurable disease that "lays waste to muscles while leaving the mind intact." Patients with the disease "typically live no more than four years after the onset of symptoms," but the exact amount of time can vary. Last summer, after a bout of pneumonia, Dr. Wesley's physician determined that he "most likely had only six months to live." Because of the Death with Dignity Act in his home state of Washington, Dr. Wesley was able to obtain a prescription for life-ending barbiturates. When asked at what point he would consider taking them, Dr. Wesley replied, "It's like the definition of pornography, I'll know it . . . when I see it."[3]

The point here is not to make any judgments about the propriety or desirability of such deaths but rather to draw attention to the prevalence and kind of human agency enacted in them. In very different ways, each case illustrates the tendency of modern medicine to bring the nature and timing of death and dying under efficient and instrumental control. In the first case, the agency displayed was not so much Mrs. Carver's as it was her family and physicians'. Once upon a time, pneumonia (the "old person's friend") may have meant a relatively peaceful passing for Mrs. Carver. In this case, it occasioned a costly series of interventions aimed at forestalling eventual death. Although the cause of her death was technically her underlying disease, once the momentum of treatment began, death could not occur until a positive decision was made by the physicians to step out of the way.

In the second case, it is the patient whose agency comes to the fore. Dr. Wesley would "prefer to die naturally, but if dying becomes protracted and difficult, he plans to take the drugs and die peacefully within minutes." Of course, suicide has always been an option for those who face the possibility of suffering. The novelty here lies in the fact that Dr. Wesley's suicide has been incorporated into the basic standard of care for persons in his position. In his home state, it has been determined that a request for life-ending drugs should be granted by a licensed physician if patients like Dr. Wesley meet certain criteria. Of course, instances of physician-assisted suicide (PAS)[4] are still relatively rare in the United States, but if the experiences of the Netherlands, Switzerland, and Canada are indicative, it is reasonable to expect a significant increase over time.[5]

These cases, chosen nearly at random from a host of possible examples, illustrate what it looks like for death and dying to be gradually drawn into the sphere of human agency and ipso facto into the sphere of moral responsibility. They also indicate the sense of moral confusion and ambiguity that can be associated with such responsibility. This change—death moving into the realm of human agency—and its implications brings with it the ethical phenomenon I call burdened agency. As we shall see, burdened agency arises through a confluence of novel medical technologies, commercial and bureaucratic forces, the radical prioritization of individualism, the proliferation of choice, and other deep social-structural changes characteristic of modernity.[6]

In introducing the concept of burdened agency, I emphasize two elements of the contemporary situation. First, there is a tendency for the *availability* of control over some aspects of the dying process to become an (often unwelcome) *imperative to make choices* that directly affect when and how death will occur—whether through living wills and advance directives, decisions to withdraw treatment, or pursuing physician-assisted suicide or euthanasia. This includes, but goes beyond, the simple fact that more and more control over the dying process is possible than ever before. That, in and of itself, could not credibly be described as a burden. Rather, it is the unsought-for nature of the agency that makes it potentially burdensome. This is the burden *of* agency itself, a gradual shift in the human relationship with death from the passive to the active voice.

The question of whether such control, or responsibility, is desirable or not is a complex one. Certainly, underprivileged and marginalized populations lacking access to adequate health care could protest that their burden lies precisely in their *lack* of agency.[7] Furthermore, many patients in fact desire, and at times demand, the maximum amount of control over the conditions of their care near the end of life. Nevertheless, the central issue of burdened agency in not unique to a particular social class, race, or gender, though it will be distinctively filtered through these elements of identity and social location.[8] Indeed, it seems to me that the disparities that exist along the lines of race and class actually *amplify* the experience of burdened agency. For example, those from less privileged segments of society are likely to have disproportionately low access to *preventative* health care, to experience unjust conditions of social determinants of health, to have lower levels of health literacy, and to receive less clinical attention or face-to-face time with physicians.[9] Yet, under these conditions, they are still faced with difficult health-care decisions at the end of life, especially as technological medicine and clinical research trials are integrated into Medicare reimbursement policies.[10] To make such decisions under the conditions of poverty, sexism, institutional racism, and mistrust is to bear an *additional* burden on one's agency. For now, it is enough to note that the shift I am describing will, at the very least, *feel* burdensome to many people to the degree that such novel decisions are morally complicated and existentially fraught for those who have to make them.

In addition to this first sense of burdening, the burden of having to choose, there is a second way in which moral agency is burdened. This aspect may be called the burden of *reflexivity*, by which I mean the added strain of making such choices in the absence of guiding social, cultural, or religious norms. It has often been noted that in premodern and early modern societies, the experience of dying was thoroughly ensconced in communal systems of meaning, which prescribed recognizable and largely predictable patterns of behavior. In our own day, no longer guided by norms that are taken for granted, individuals are, more or less, left to self-consciously negotiate the experience of dying on their own. To describe modern agency as burdened, then, is also to highlight the way these decisions seem to labor under the existential "weight" of ambiguity, instability, and uncertainty that accompany highly reflexive moral action.

In short, human agency, once largely considered to be passive in the face of death, is increasingly asked to take control of the conditions of dying—at the very moment that the social institutions that could provide guidance for such agency are gradually fragmenting. We live under a paradox. On the one hand, death has never been more strange and more foreign to human experience. On the other hand, modern medicine succeeds in placing the conditions of our dying directly into human hands. How to cope with this responsibility in an age of moral confusion is an important task for a rapidly aging population.

Some who are reading this may be wondering about the relationship my concept of burdened agency has with Lisa Tessman's concept of burdened virtues. Although the two terms are not essentially related (I am not drawing directly on Tessman's work here), there are certain resonances between the two concepts. Tessman offers a picture of virtue formation that acknowledges and accepts the effects of moral luck. In doing so, she challenges Aristotle's contention that the exercise of virtues must be constitutively and essentially related to human flourishing. For Tessman, even a virtuous person under the conditions of oppression will sometimes exhibit "burdened virtues, virtues that have the unusual feature of being disjoined from their bearer's own flourishing,"[11] something not thought possible by Aristotle. For example, an oppressed woman may be morally correct in showing "the kind of anger that would normally be quite wrong but that under the extraordinary conditions of oppression are actually morally recommended."[12] Such an act will be accompanied by a feeling of "agent-regret . . . [as she] takes at least partial responsibility despite lack of complete control"[13] over her situation. Often enough, given conditions of oppression and moral damage, the morally prescribed action will, if taken, lead to inner turmoil and conflict (similar to Aristotle's conception of the "pain" that accompanies acts of continence). My own concept "burdened agency" shares this sense of inner turmoil and even regret. It is also similar in that agency, like virtue, is normally considered to be an unambiguous good, but I hope to show, as Tessman has, that agency (as it is widely conceived) is not *necessarily* ingredient to one's well-being and flourishing. One difference between our accounts lies in my characterization of burdened agency as a typical feature of modernity rather than a constitutive aspect of moral life as such.

To forestall an obvious objection to what follows, let me be perfectly clear at the outset that nothing in what follows should be taken as a rejection of modern medicine, which is the source of innumerable benefits to humankind. Modern medicine has expanded not only the average human life span but also the average number of healthy years. On the whole, people today live longer, healthier lives than ever before. When I speak about coping with the problem of burdened agency, I do not mean to imply that the solution should be the *unburdening* of agency, if by that is meant a return to premodern forms of dying or a wholesale rejection of life-prolonging medical technology. I consider that both impossible and undesirable. Nevertheless, an appreciation for the benefits we enjoy should not preclude an honest investigation of the moral ambiguities and challenges of our situation. Such an investigation is the first step in addressing the particular challenges we face. It is to this task that I now turn.

DYING BEFORE MODERNITY

To truly understand how profound the burden of agency is, one must understand the rapid growth of medical technologies over the past two centuries. More important, however, one must also understand the gradual change in cultural assumptions about the nature of the body, its susceptibility to human control, the extent to which medicine might be expected to intervene in the dying process, and the influence of advanced capitalism and the pervasive consumer ethos to which it gives rise.

The physician Sherwin Nuland once noted that "every scientific or clinical advance carries with it a cultural implication, and often a symbolic one."[14] Naturally, advances in medical technology change the way we die, but arguably more important are the deeper assumptions that accompany the development and use of these technologies—assumptions, for example, about the nature of the body, the place of sickness and death in a good human life, and the question of the limits of human control. These not only affect the material conditions but also the existential and psychological experience of our dying. Moreover, cultural assumptions feed back to influence the development and use of new technologies and new institutional structures that provide the context for human experience.[15]

Perhaps the most widely cited historical study on death and dying, Philippe Ariès's *The Hour of Our Death*, makes the claim that dying was once "tame" and has now become "wild." He gives the following example of a tame death: "In 1874, [Madame Pouget] contracted a summer cholera. After four days she asked to see the village priest, who came and wanted to give her the last rites. 'Not yet, Monsieur le Cure; I'll let you know when the time comes.' Two days later: 'Go and tell Monsieur le Cure to bring me Extreme Unction.'"[16] In this very short anecdote, there are two discernable elements of a tame death: "familiar simplicity" and a "public" or, perhaps better, "social" nature.[17] In what sense was Madame Pouget's death familiar or simple? For Ariès, "familiarity" refers both to the fact that people were more likely to encounter dead and dying people during their lives and to the fact that they were more likely to know what to do when such encounters occurred. Madame Pouget's was a death forewarned by physical symptoms, "which initiated a 'ritual moment' of preparation for dying . . . [a] highly social, choreographed event."[18] Daniel Callahan notes the considerable advantage of such familiarity in "the comfort of knowing how to behave publicly in the presence of death—what to say, how to compose one's face, to whom to speak, and when to speak."[19]

In addition to making death familiar, ritual also made it social. When death seemed imminent, the dying person would gather his or her children and family around the bed and would offer final instructions and farewells. According to Ariès, such a death was "always public. . . . The dying person must be the center of a group of people."[20] With the priest present, the dying person would perform various rites, such as "the profession of faith, the confession of sins, the pardon of the survivors, the pious dispositions on their behalf, the commendation of one's soul to God, [and] the choice of burial."[21] In the late Middle Ages, these practices were compiled in wildly popular pamphlets called *ars moriendi*, which instructed lay Christians in the etiquette of proper dying.[22] This liturgy completed, the dying person would simply wait for death to arrive, as would the family members and friends who were able to do so. "All of this prescribed activity [took] place at the bedside, preferably in a crowded room filled with onlookers" who would thereby receive a good example for their own dying.[23]

In contrast to this "tame death," what medieval people feared above all was a sudden or secret death. To die suddenly or in isolation "was a vile and ugly death; it was frightening. It seemed a strange and monstrous thing that nobody dared talk about."[24] Such a frightening prospect, according to Ariès, has now become the norm. Death in the hospital, as we shall see below, is often lonely, secret, alien, and unwieldy—in short, "wild." Its wildness stems from its asociality.

It might be argued that death in the modern hospital is characteristically *more* public than a death in the home, for there is a greater chance that one will die in front of a group of people. One thinks of the steady stream of nurses, medical students, residents, and specialists that are likely to cycle through one's hospital room on any given day. But death in front of strangers is, for all practical purposes, as solitary as a death in isolation. It is not the mere presence of other people that makes death social but the nature of one's relationship to those others. The relevant relationships are characterized by personal relations and affective bonds, rather than impersonal norms based on market or bureaucratic forces. As Wendell Berry puts it, the hospital is the place where the "world of love" and the "world of efficiency" "come together . . . but do not meet."[25] It is only the former, and not the latter, that can help to tame death.

THE ROAD TO THE ICU

The development of modern medicine entailed certain changes in the relationship between physician and patient. Consider what medicine was like in the early modern period. First, for those who could afford it, medical care took place almost exclusively in the home of either the physician or of the patient. Second, the primary technique for medical diagnosis was personal narrative, with observation and physical examination following only in necessary cases. Because of standards of decorum, physical touch would be limited, especially when patients were women. Sometimes, to avoid difficult travel, physicians would diagnose illnesses and prescribe treatment through the mail, based on the written first-person account offered by the ailing patient.

New approaches to medical diagnosis altered this relationship. For the most part, the changes were subtle, but on the whole, they constituted a cumulative effect. Parting ways with the medieval medical theory of humors, physicians gradually adopted a theory of anatomically localized pathology. According to the emerging anatomical view, diseases reside in particular bodily tissues. Therefore, the best way to diagnose an illness is through a direct physical examination of the diseased area, initially, for example, through a method called "'percussion'—striking the body with the fingers to produce sounds indicating the vitality of underlying organs."[26] A further change occurred with the invention of the stethoscope in 1816. This introduced a mechanical intermediary "by which physicians came to distance themselves from their patients."[27] Moreover, the stethoscope brought the physician into a world of sounds that the patient herself could not hear.

The trajectory of technological alienation between physician and patient continued throughout the nineteenth century. The invention of the ophthalmoscope, laryngoscope, and X-ray machine allowed physicians for the first time to peer into the human body without having to cut it open. Sight, once again, began to eclipse sound, but the observation process now took place *technologically*. X-ray, especially, changed the method of examination. With the X-ray, the physician no longer needed the patient in front of him or her to carry out an evaluation of the disease. The development of the microscope, which led to advances in cellular pathology and bacteriology, also aided in making the patient's presence unnecessary; all that was needed was a sample of some bodily tissue or fluid from the patient. As historian Stanley Reiser suggests, the depersonalization of medicine is perhaps nowhere more apparent than with the development of statistical medicine in the late nineteenth century: "The conversion of physiological signals generated by respiration, circulation, and heat production, into graphs and numbers, allowed physicians to obtain clear and accurate records . . . to free these signals from the limitation of private analysis . . . and open them to group inquiry; to make them objective and invest them with unambiguous meanings that were evident to all physicians."[28]

The estrangement of the patient from the physician occurred alongside of, and probably encouraged, a changing view of the human body. Jeffrey Bishop argues that such changes amounted to the body's objectification and mechanization. Bishop argues that modern medicine came to see the body as "matter in motion" because its epistemology was grounded in the "decontextualized dead body"—specifically the dissection cadaver used in medical education.[29] Bishop draws attention to Michel Foucault's work on the rise of "discourse" in medicine through a separation of the symptom (the subjective experience of a disease) from the sign (the objectively verifiable and observable indication of a disease). According to Foucault, this shift placed the patient under the "penetrating gaze" of the physician, who now applied analytical techniques to decipher the signs of disease.[30] Bishop extends Foucault's account by explicitly connecting the physician's gaze with the early adoption of the practice of postmortem autopsy: "the techniques of the clinic elicited what could only have been known definitively through dissection of the body. The analytic technique acts in the same manner as the autopsy. Both reveal disease; the violence of the penetrating gaze is an analogue to the violence of opening the corpse. The new normative object, the dead body, comes to represent the patient's living body, claims Foucault. The patient, who was the absolute subject of the disease, *has now become the object* against which both the gaze and the analytic probing of the doctor are now directed."[31]

Of course, in reality, human bodies are dynamic. They are constantly and unpredictably changing and are therefore insufficient foundations for a form of scientific knowledge that stresses reproducibility and measurability. With the autopsy, medical professionals believed that they had discovered a static, observable, manipulable, and measurable object of study: the dead body. The truth, of course, is that the body is never static, not even in death.

This is important because the myth of the dead body as the stable foundation for medical knowledge encouraged "certain notions of causation over others and deploy[ed] practices that shape, direct, and enforce what we call care."[32] Specifically, it encouraged an understanding of "life" as a "series of functions that resist death."[33] Sustaining life, on this view, is a matter of intervening in prior efficient causes, typically by replacing the failing body part with an artificial or donated substitute. It's easy to see how this understanding of life encouraged a mechanistic understanding of the body and of medicine.

THE ICU AND THE BURDEN *OF* AGENCY

The ICU epitomizes the success of technological interventions and points to the importance of the preceding story for understanding the contemporary burden *of* agency. In the ICU, "life" can, in many cases, be sustained almost indefinitely. This mechanical prolonging of bare life strikes many as a fate worse than death, but as we saw with the case of Mrs. Carver, modern medicine typically lacks the internal resources to put the brakes on.

In fact, treatment in the ICU is often governed, in an apt phrase coined by philosopher Daniel Callahan, by the logic of "technological brinkmanship." Callahan notes, "There has been a powerful clinical drive to push technology as far as possible to save life while, at the same time, preserving a decent quality of life. It is well recognized by now that, if medical technology is pushed too far, a person can be harmed, that there is a line that should not be crossed. I define 'brinkmanship' as the gambling effort to go *as close to that line as possible* before the cessation or abatement of treatment."[34]

To mitigate the effects of such brinkmanship, "medicine's response is to create the patient as the master of her own body. She *must decide* whether to embrace or reject technology."[35] Accordingly, landmark cases in the early history of bioethics focused on patients' rights to deny life-prolonging treatments. Such "right to die" cases focused public attention on the difficult task of opposing the inertia of technological medicine. They also firmly established in public consciousness the overwhelming importance and centrality of respect for patient autonomy.

Of course, as highly publicized incidents like the Terri Schiavo case make clear, the patient may not be capable of making decisions at the end of life. This is increasingly the case for a growing population of persons experiencing dementia or dementia-like symptoms. There are complicated questions surrounding such surrogate decisions. What qualifications are necessary for someone to serve as a surrogate decision maker? Are family members better suited to fulfill this role than health professionals or "impartial" advisers (e.g., hospital ethics committees or judges)? On what sort of criteria should such decisions be made? What role should a patient's previously stated desires and values play? Can they be overridden by judgments about a patient's current best interests? What role should quality-of-life judgments play and what are the relevant criteria for making such evaluations? What if there are disagreements among family members or between family members and health-care professionals?

Given these complexities, it is no wonder that there has been a strong push for the adoption and use of advance directives (sometimes called a living will). With an advance directive, a person takes the opportunity, while still competent, to specify in writing her preferences for treatment in the event that she should become incompetent, including specifying which medical treatments she would prefer to forgo given the presence of relevant circumstances (e.g., "In the event that I am determined to be in a permanent vegetative state, all medical life-sustaining treatments shall be withdrawn"). A common motivation for adopting a living will is the desire to avoid burdening loved ones with the responsibility for making difficult decisions, especially about the withdrawal of life-sustaining treatments. Unfortunately, advance directives are a notoriously ineffective means of guiding such decisions. In the all-too-likely event that a living will fails to apply to a given situation, the designated proxy decision maker may be faced with the prospect of balancing judgments about what a patient *would have wanted* with judgments about *what is best* for her now. Surrogates often suffer from psychological distress. Furthermore, in highly stressful situations, where the knowledge and power differential between physicians and patients or surrogates is great, it is not always easy to determine where the agency of the physician ends and that of the patient or surrogate begins.

One thing, however, is clear: when "death [becomes] a medically-timed phenomenon,"[36] *someone* will be making a decision. As medical anthropologist Sharon Kaufman notes, "Hospital treatment and hospital logic work to prolong life, stave off dying, and then *make death happen.*"[37] Increasingly, the manner and timing of one's death is a matter of deliberation and choice.

THE LOSS OF CULTURAL APTITUDE

Blaise Pascal once remarked that we all die alone. The irony of the aphorism depends on it being figuratively true but not literally true. Today, the statement has been turned into a truism. In contrast to previous ages, death in the hospital or nursing home, at least in modern-day America, is often a solitary affair.

How did this happen? The rise of the hospital is one key factor. Originating from late-medieval charitable houses, early hospitals sought to extend an explicitly Christian notion of *hospitalitas* to those in need.[38] But hospitals necessarily changed with the development of novel diagnostic and therapeutic tools and the rapid increase in *specialization* of medicine at the turn of the twentieth century. No single person could any longer have comprehensive knowledge of all anatomical and pathological data or be expected to know how to use all the newest medical instruments. Soon, the need was felt to organize physicians with different specialties into "cooperative practices." In urban areas, such centralization led to the formation of large hospitals and private practices, which were increasingly commercialized and bureaucratized.

There is a correlation between the physical isolation of the dying and a broader cultural discomfort with death and dying. Already in the mid-1950s, Geoffrey Gorer noticed a contradictory impulse in modern Western attitudes toward death and dying. In an essay titled "The Pornography of Death," Gorer likened the predominant view of death to the Victorian attitude toward sexuality: simultaneously obsessive and repressive, fascinated but unwilling to speak of it. It was this curious combination that led Gorer to call death the modern "taboo."[39]

Indeed, multiple studies conducted during this period showed that most physicians refused to mention a patient's terminal cancer diagnosis, even if they had reason to believe the patient already had knowledge about the diagnosis from another source.[40] Of course, this would strike most of us as an outrageous affront to patient autonomy, which shows how far attitudes have come. But this does not mean that open discussions about death are commonplace, even in a medical context. Between 1989 and 1994, researchers conducting the Study to Understand Prognoses and Preferences for Outcomes and Risks of Treatments (SUPPORT) demonstrated a severe lack of understanding of patient preferences on the part of physicians, as well as a higher-than-expected prevalence of pain and suffering in the last days of patients' lives. According to Dr. Joanne Lynn, one of the researchers, "The problem was much more difficult than that doctors did not hear their patients' requests; it was that no one involved was talking about these subjects."[41] In fact, more recent studies indicate that patients and physicians engage in a mutual process of active collusion to avoid talking about death and dying.[42]

Sociologist Anthony Giddens notes a modern tendency to shield "day-to-day life from contact with experiences which raise potentially disturbing existential questions—particularly experiences to do with sickness, madness, criminality, sexuality, and death."[43] The effect of such "sequestration" "means that for many people, direct contact with events and situations which link the individual lifespan to broad issues of mortality and finitude are rare and fleeting."[44] As a result, many people's understanding of illness and death is filtered through popular media (novels, movies, video games, etc.) rather than direct experience. Such "experience," needless to say, does not lead to the sort of familiarity with death that Ariès claims is typical of premodern societies but rather to a false, abstract, and sensationalized familiarity. The modern confusion and awkwardness surrounding social interaction in hospital rooms and funeral parlors is an example of what happens when death is consistently hidden from sight. As always, the Germans have a handy term for this: *Handlungsverlust*, the loss of the capacity to act. The resulting sense of inadequacy impedes social interactions and further motivates us to shield death from view. No one likes having awkward conversations.

Beginning in the 1960s, scholarly attention began turning toward the issues Gorer had diagnosed. Works by Jessica Mitford, Herman Feifel, Elisabeth Kübler-Ross, and others resulted in an emergent "death awareness movement."[45] Largely as a result of this movement, it is no longer possible to claim that death is "taboo" in quite the same way that it was when Gorer first published his essay. Hospice and palliative care medicine, which stress openness and transparency between physicians and patients, have enjoyed growing success since their advent in the 1960s and are now firmly within the mainstream of medical care. College courses on death and dying from a variety of disciplinary perspectives are common today. Television shows and films focusing on themes of death and dying enjoy broad popular appeal. Books and memoirs about death and dying regularly become bestsellers.[46] Today, a small but growing number of people are even hosting "death cafés"—small, intimate gatherings that aim "to increase awareness of death with a view to helping people make the most of their (finite) lives."[47]

These curious phenomena indicate a somewhat surprising openness surrounding issues of death and dying in contemporary culture. Nevertheless, it would be a mistake to conclude that most people are now comfortable talking about death or, even less, being around those who are dying. The dying are all too often institutionalized and separated from meaningful interactions with others. For example, medical anthropologist Jennifer Hockey demonstrates how the nursing home functions as a "zone of social abandonment."[48] All too often, the regrettable effect of the isolation of the aged is an accelerated decline of emotional and physical health—a paradigm instance of what Ivan Illich calls "specific diseconomy" or "counterproductivity."[49] It is as if in the attempt to forestall and evade death, modern medicine ironically leads to a condition that prematurely mirrors the negative effects of death—namely, alienation from our bodies and communities.

HYPERREFLEXIVE DYING

In the handy, if inelegant, parlance of cultural sociology, death and dying has become "hyperreflexive" as a result of *deinstitutionalization*. This claim relies on a specific theory of institutions, developed by sociologists Peter Berger and Thomas Luckmann. These authors argue that the roots of human culture are related to human physiology and development. The human being at birth is in a uniquely dependent position. Both physically and instinctually, the newborn is underdeveloped and premature.[50] All other animals live in "closed worlds," meaning that almost all of their interactions with the world are predetermined by an instinctual apparatus calibrated to a species-specific environment. "By contrast, man's [sic] relationship to his environment is characterized by world-openness. . . . His relationship to the surrounding environment is everywhere very imperfectly structured by his own biological constitution."[51] Human beings suffer, we might say, from instinctual-deficit disorder.

Human life is fundamentally open-ended and therefore unstable. If humans had to operate solely based on biological and instinctual resources, the result would be anomic chaos. To provide a stable environment for human life, human beings rely on habitual, communally recognized norms of action. These norms are created by society (externalization) before they are experienced as an objective reality (objectivation) and subsequently shape the next generation (internalization). Through this process, human beings fill the gap left by instinctual deprivation and give the world a sense of meaning and intelligibility that allows them to get on with the business of living. Berger and Luckmann refer to this process as "institutionalization" and the norms that perform this function as "institutions."[52]

Institutions, in this very particular sense of the term, remove certain existential threats from the *foreground* of human experience (i.e., that part about which we think, ponder, and deliberate) and place them in the *background* (i.e., that part that may be taken for granted). Anthony Giddens has written about how this backgrounding, or "bracketing," provides human beings with a sense of "*ontological security*."[53] According to Giddens, one of the defining marks of humanity is "reflexive awareness," the ability to know "both what one is doing and why one is doing it."[54] This ability is an asset to humanity, but if left unchecked, it can be potentially overwhelming. Were we unable to bracket out an almost infinite number of possible considerations, we would be overwhelmed by anxiety and unable to function. "To be ontologically secure is to possess, on the level of the unconscious and practical consciousness, 'answers' to fundamental existential questions which all human life in some way addresses."[55] Institutions, in Berger's sense, aid in the development of practical consciousness by providing channels by which we can move much of life out of the reflexive sphere (foreground) and into the taken-for-granted sphere (background).

According to Berger, institutions bear a special relationship to death and dying: "every human society is, in the last resort, men banded together in the face of death."[56] If the overriding effect of sociality is to give the individual a sense of meaning that has the force of instinct, then one of the greatest threats to the individual is meaninglessness. The marginal situations in life challenge the sheltering quality of the social order and threaten the individual with "unbearable psychological tensions." Death, according to Berger, is "the marginal situation *par excellence*." Death causes us to question the ad hoc nature of our social ordering and thereby challenges the very foundation of our shared institutions by putting "in question the taken-for-granted, 'business-as-usual' attitude in which one exists in everyday life." Because death is an unavoidable aspect of life, "legitimations of the reality of the social world *in the face of death* are decisive requirements in any society." What is at stake here is not simply social control but *reality* itself—that is, the power of the social apparatus to "constitute and to impose itself as reality." Historically, the dominant institution that made such legitimation possible was religion. The religiously defined "good death" placed even this most marginal situation in the context of a meaningful story of the human world.

Notably, this means that some amount of death "denial" is a normal, and probably necessary, aspect of the human condition. This was the argument of Ernest Becker, who followed Sigmund Freud and Otto Rank in arguing that death denial was at the root of all human culture.[57] Because humans are unique in their awareness of their vulnerability, fragility, and ultimate mortality, they uniquely experience anxiety about finitude. It isn't so much that we are afraid of dying at any particular moment, but our generalized sense of dread is ultimately linked to our vulnerability and mortality. To escape the anxiety this awareness produces in us, we devise cultural strategies of avoidance. We invest our being in projects that aim at permanence or that we invest with ultimate meaning.[58]

Dying is increasingly *deinstitutionalized* in North Atlantic societies. Two things follow from this. First, the onus for meaning making is shifted to individuals. Charles Taylor calls this aspect "subjectivation."[59] When one looks to institutions for meaning, identity, or guidance and they do not provide stable answers, then one may be forced to look inward.[60] Second, one is faced with what Giddens calls the "routine contemplation of counterfactuals"[61] in almost every domain of human life. In other words, the modern condition entails the loss of the "taken for granted" and the resulting ascendancy of hyperreflexive awareness. As a result, we are now faced with the *foregrounding* of experiences like death and dying.

Because this description of hyperreflexive awareness is central for my claim that contemporary dying has an additional burdened quality beyond the sheer proliferation of choice itself, it is important to consider a possible objection. It might reasonably be asked whether what I am describing as deinstitutionalization would not better be described in terms of death and dying being "differently institutionalized." If human life is inherently cultural, it would seem unlikely—barring extreme, nay apocalyptic, circumstances—that we could thrust off cultural institutions altogether. To be sure, the institutions that once were dominant are no longer dominant, but this does not leave us bereft of institutions themselves. What institutions now envelop the dying process today?

Two major candidates are (a) the institution of research medicine, including biomedical technology and "Big Pharma," which is growing at an exponential rate, and (b) advanced global capitalism, which threatens to turn all relationships into market relationships and which emphasizes individual choice to the highest degree possible. These two institutions, the objection continues, effectively order our choices, doing so in a manner that is largely taken for granted—a hallmark of strong institutions. We are often unaware of the deep logics that are guiding our decisions, often before we ever come to the point of decision. This occurs partly through the "choice architecture" that precedes our choosing and is the result of innumerable decisions of others (some organic and unintentional, some premeditated to guide you to a predetermined end). It also occurs through repeated exposure to the logics of research medicine and market rationality (reinforced by the social status and "capital" enjoyed by these institutions), which convey particular understandings of agency and selfhood.

Perhaps, then, it would be better to give a more fine-grained account of the institutions that exist in the background of our modern moral agency. To this I counter that the institutions of research medicine and market capitalism differ *in kind* from the previous sort because they are inherently destabilizing. They are what sociologist Zygmunt Bauman would call "liquid" rather than "solid" institutions.[62] For all its flaws, I retain the notion of deinstitutionalization because the term signifies the foregrounding of moral agency through the "routine contemplation of counterfactuals" (Giddens). To the degree that research medicine and market capitalism are the institutions that predominate today (they very much are), they gain their power by *liquidizing* meaning-making reference groups. They destabilize cultures and societies, typically toward the end of convincing us that we need to purchase some good or service to become more secure. They make us into *homo arbitrius*: "man, the chooser."

CONCLUSION: BEARING BURDENED AGENCY

As a result of both increased technological capacities and decreased institutional norms, death in modernity is increasingly a hyperreflexive project, a matter of deliberation and choice. This manifests itself in the many choices to be made when death occurs in the ICU: Should life-sustaining treatment be withheld or withdrawn? Should a patient be kept on life support to hold open the possibility of a miracle recovery? Should suffering be avoided at all costs? Can death ever be directly intended? Is terminal sedation ever a viable option? Should the family sign a DNR (do not resuscitate) order? Should health-care providers urge surrogates to complete one against their initial judgment? In the event that the family refuses, can health-care workers perform a "slow code" to prevent treatment, which is likely to be as futile and potentially damaging as Mrs. Carver's? It is also reflected in the many positive decisions that must be made to *avoid* death in the ICU. Even after someone has been placed in home hospice care, it is not uncommon for her to end up dying in the hospital. Hospice nurses and physicians often must urge home caretakers to call them instead of emergency services, for a knee-jerk 911 call will undo previous efforts to enable a home death.

The number of choices at the end of life, and the nature of these choices, is often experienced as an uninvited burden *of* agency. Because most people involved (whether patients, surrogates, or medical professionals) seem to have inadequate resources to bear this burden, the lack of cultural guidance is experienced as an added burden *on* that agency. Where once there were liturgies for dying, we are now thrown back on our own resources. Unhinged from strong institutions of family and church, sequestered in private hospital rooms, and shielded from public view, these decisions are often made in a highly subjective manner, often accompanied by considerable existential anxiety and moral confusion. It is not clear that we have the resources to deal with the forms of agency we are increasingly asked to enact: we feel burdened by agency and we feel that our agency itself labors under the strain of a dizzying anomie. In this context, it might seem that the only thing left to do is to take control, to embrace responsibility, and shape our dying according to our preferences as best we can.

On the other hand, we cannot, *ultimately*, control death. Most of us implicitly understand that death signals the absolute limit of any human pursuit of control. This is why our situation presents us with a *false sense of agency*. We increasingly feel that we must control death, but ultimately, death comes to each of us as something beyond our control. There is something profoundly sad about the false dichotomies presented to the patient with an incurable, terminal illness. Should the patient with stage-five metastatic cancer "keep fighting," or would it be better to just "give up"? Can we plausibly conclude that someone has "given up" on life when she chooses not to pursue a fourth-line chemotherapy regime with known side effects and only a marginal chance of success? The unfortunate irony of burdened agency is that this is sometimes experienced as "choosing to die" even when it comes at the end of a series of aggressive medical treatments.

Our agency, then, is burdened twice over: once by choices and once by what I have called reflexivity. Both of these forms of burdened agency coalesce in the ICU, where technology succeeds in placing decisions about the nature and timing of dying directly in human hands. This endowment of responsibility all too often results in an awkward attempt to toe the line between appropriate life extension and overly medicalized dying—an attitude of technological brinkmanship shared by doctors, patients, and surrogates alike.

This is not a situation that admits of easy, quick fixes. There is no going back to a premodern form of dying. We are unlikely as a society to stop utilizing life-extending technologies that place us in the position of having to choose between life and death. We are also unlikely to reverse the deep cultural dynamics of pluralization and secularization that have helped to unhinge dying from the cultural forms typical of the *ars moriendi*.

Where, then, do we go from here? Are there any resources that might allow us to make some headway toward a good and appropriate form of dying within the conditions of modern society and medicine? I believe there are, but I also believe they will have to come from outside of the current mainstream of medicine and biomedical ethics. Death, dying, and mortality bring us to the edge of human experience, provoking questions of meaning that cannot be answered from within the imminent frame of modern scientific rationality. In chapter 3 I will therefore turn to religious and theological views of death and dying, restricting my purview to the Christian tradition. I hope in doing so to bring to light theological themes (sometimes underappreciated ones) that might energize faith communities in their efforts to grapple with the choices with which they are likely to be burdened, especially in an aging and technological society such as ours. The theological themes in chapters 3–6 build up to suggest an alternative framework for understanding the shape of moral agency. Taken together, these deeply challenge predominant cultural assumptions and social practices at the end of life.

But first, I must delve a bit deeper into the landscape of modern dying. I have here highlighted a puzzling dynamic at the heart of our current end-of-life practices. This dynamic has to do with the mismatch between our deep-seated assumptions about the nature of human moral agency and the experience of that agency at the end of life. This tension is not merely incidental. It is rooted in a complex series of ideals, beliefs, and expectations that define for us, largely pre-reflectively, what we consider to be the ideal forms of human moral agency. It is to the relationship between what Charles Taylor has called "modern social imaginaries" and the conflicts of modern dying that we now turn.

TWO

Scripts for Dying

HOSPICE OR HEMLOCK?

Most of us would prefer not to die in the intensive care unit (ICU). It is, however, often surprisingly difficult to avoid that fate. In our current medical culture, new technologies carry a certain amount of inertia into our deliberations about their use. Especially as they are incorporated into our sense of ordinary medicine and are covered by major insurers like Medicare, life-prolonging technologies are often employed pell-mell. Unless previous thought has been given to the suitability of their use, the very existence of a technology capable of extending human life is taken as sufficient justification for its implementation.

We live and die in a context that is increasingly marked by burdened agency. This means that dying increasingly is a hyperreflexive project of the individual self. Part of the problem is the lack of cultural guidance that might otherwise provide moral norms and shape our attitudes toward dying. And yet, it would be wrong to conclude that there are *no* available cultural scripts. Indeed, two prominent responses have arisen as responses to burdened agency: hospice and palliative care, on the one hand, and physician-assisted suicide (PAS) and euthanasia, on the other. These, according to Michael Banner, constitute our two "scripts" for dying—the two most culturally visible pathways to dying.¹ Or, as the title of another monograph indicates, if we desire to avoid the ICU, we are forced to make our decision between "Hospice or Hemlock."²

But why *these* particular scripts? This chapter explores the cultural currents that inform both hospice and assisted suicide as ascending cultural frameworks for dying. The scripts we inherit are always value laden, carrying forward certain deeply held (often invisible and pre-reflective) moral norms. The work of philosopher Charles Taylor illustrates how each of these scripts is deeply rooted in what he calls the "modern identity" though in different ways and with different emphases. My goal is to highlight the implicit norms of these social practices to open them up to the possibility of rational self-criticism and to engagement with alternative frameworks from within the Christian theological tradition.

Hospice and palliative care medicine are commonly associated with each other, but they refer to slightly different practices. In general, "palliative care" refers to any medical care whose primary goal is the relief of suffering. The palliative care philosophy can be summed up in the aphorism, "To cure sometimes, to relieve often, to comfort always." It is sometimes assumed that palliative care represents a departure from conventional medicine, a point that most palliative care physicians would reject. Rather, they would contend that palliative care and conventional medicine are part of an integrated continuum of care. The former is not distinguished from the latter because it seeks a *mutually exclusive* goal (e.g., care rather than cure) but by a "strong emphasis on specific principles, such as alleviation of suffering, symptom management, good communication, and supportive counseling related to illness, disability, and limited prognosis."³ Advocates of this approach believe there is no reason why palliative care should not begin at the "diagnosis of progressive incurable illness or any constellation of medical problems that result in progressive disability or an *eventually* terminal prognosis."⁴ Palliative medicine focuses on increasing the quality of life of all such patients, even if they are receiving treatments (from other specialists) aimed at curing their illness.

Hospice care, on the other hand, departs more fully from conventional medicine's curative goals. The modern hospice movement began when

Dame Cicely Saunders helped to found St. Christopher's Hospice in 1967. A religiously inspired response to the inadequate care given to incurable terminally ill patients, Saunders sought to address the "total pain" (physical, emotional, social, and spiritual) of dying persons. Hospice care incorporates palliative concepts along with communal practices to ensure that no patient dies alone or in pain. Limited to situations in which the person is approaching death (usually defined as a prognosis of less than six months to live), hospice involves a recognition that curative therapy is no longer appropriate, because such treatment is not clinically indicated, is overly burdensome, or is no longer desired by the patient.

Hospice seeks to avoid overly medicalized death. This same impulse is shared by proponents of PAS and euthanasia. Advocates of PAS often rely on narratives of bad deaths—deaths laden with inescapable pain and suffering despite the application of every available curative technology and/or pharmaceutical palliative measure—to encourage a shift in cultural attitudes toward voluntary ending of life.[5] The message is clear: to die well, you must be empowered to die on your own terms. According to recent Gallup polls, 72 percent of Americans now support euthanasia, with much of the increased support coming from eighteen- to thirty-four-year-olds, an increase of 24 percent over a two-year span and the highest level in more than a decade.[6] The increasing awareness of PAS in the public imagination is paralleled by increasing recourse to PAS in states where it is an available option. Although accurate statistics are sometimes difficult to come by (largely due to underreporting of PAS in states that prohibit it), it does seem that the availability of PAS leads to more frequent occurrences. In Oregon, for example, which has allowed PAS since 1997, there has been a slight but steady increase in both prescriptions for life-ending barbiturates and instances of PAS.[7] A similar trend is evidenced in Washington, which has reached near equal figures in the years since the program was instituted.[8]

Statistics reveal a much more drastic trend in Canada, where recourse to medical aid in dying, or MAID (a designation that includes both voluntary active euthanasia and physician-assisted suicide), is growing quite rapidly. According to the most recent government report, "MAID deaths accounted for 3.3% of all deaths in Canada in 2021, an increase from 2.5% in 2020 and 2.0% in 2019."[9] Indeed, MAID deaths will very soon outpace all accidental deaths in Canada and are now higher than the general suicide rate (MAID deaths are not counted as suicides under existing protocols). Furthermore, the rate of suicide has not been displaced by the increase in MAID deaths, which means that MAID is not primarily providing a gentler option for those who would otherwise commit suicide. There is a stark disparity between usage in Canada and usage in the United States. For example, despite having nearly equal populations and having legalized MAID in the same year, in 2021 in California, 486 people died using the state's assisted suicide program. In Canada in the same year, 10,064 people (a roughly twenty times higher rate) used MAID to die, even without the proposed expansion of MAID to cases involving mental illness diagnoses.

Although both hospice and PAS enjoy widespread public support, they are not without critics. Many oppose PAS on moral grounds; others fear that recourse to hospice often amounts to substandard medical care. Advocates of PAS sometimes fail to appreciate the potentially profound implications that liberalizing current laws might have on vulnerable populations, including the potential for abuse and coercion, especially for patients who are elderly and/or cognitively impaired.[10] Many advocates dismiss such concerns, claiming better regulation and enforcement can mitigate the possibility of abuse. This, however, fails to recognize what Daniel Sulmasy calls the *logical* slippery slope[11] in which the entailments of justifications for PAS lead, step by step, to policies that might not have had initial support. Begin with the claim that people have the *right* to access medical assistance in dying when faced with a terminal prognosis. If this right is legitimate, based on both poor prognosis and voluntary informed consent, then it must extend equally to similar patients who cannot self-administer the pills (someone, for example, like Dr. Wesley, who has advanced ALS). To deny such patients voluntary-active euthanasia (VAE) might be considered discriminatory.

One step further: Is the right grounded primarily in the autonomy of the patient or the attempt to prevent suffering? If the former, then is it not equally discriminatory to deny VAE in cases when the patient lacks a terminal prognosis? Consider, for example, the case of the prominent British conductor Sir Edward Thomas Downes and his wife, Lady Downes. In July 2009, the couple traveled from Great Britain to Switzerland to gain access to PAS with the assistance of the Swiss advocacy group Dignitas. Lady Downes, who was her husband's primary caretaker, was in the final stages of terminal cancer. Sir Edward, however, had no terminal diagnosis; his health was relatively stable apart from increasing blindness and hearing loss. Sir Edward, however, could not bear to live without his wife of fifty-four years. With the assistance of the advocacy group and the blessing of the couple's adult children, the two of them ingested the life-ending barbiturate and died in "adjacent beds, holding hands."[12] Cases like this demonstrate the murkiness of the moral bounds of PAS. Sadness, grief, and disability are surely regrettable circumstances, but should they be considered acceptable grounds for exercising one's *right* to assistance in dying? If the right to PAS is grounded primarily in patient autonomy—and a patient rationally and autonomously claims that a life without his beloved wife is not worth living—on what grounds *could* access be denied?

On the other hand, what if the right to PAS was grounded primarily in the compassionate relief and prevention of suffering? This may call into question whether voluntariness is an *absolutely* necessary condition. For example, consider the case of the incapacitated person. Using the standard of "substituted judgment," one may conclude that the person *would have* desired euthanasia; or using the "best interest" standard, that she *should have* desired euthanasia. Therefore, nonvoluntary active euthanasia (NAE) logically follows even though it cannot be established that the person *does* desire euthanasia. This is a similar justification that is used in the Netherlands under the Groningen Protocol, where on the basis of compassion nonvoluntary euthanasia is administered to children and infants with painful chronic diagnoses.[13]

Something very much like the logical slippery slope seems to be occurring in Canada, which is quickly becoming one of the most permissive policies in the world. MAID was originally legalized in 2016 through the passage of Bill C-14, which allowed for MAID (either self-administered or administered by a medical professional) in cases involving mentally competent adults suffering from an incurable illness whose natural death is "reasonably foreseeable." Three years later, the Superior Court of Quebec struck down the "reasonably foreseeable" clause as unconstitutional and unjust (*Truchon v. Attorney General of Canada*).

In 2021, a new law, Bill C-7, was passed, which aimed at further expanding access to MAID. The law removed the existing ten-day waiting period, the requirement to offer palliative care, and the requirement to have two independent witnesses for patients whose death is reasonably foreseeable.

It also created a path for patients whose death is not reasonably foreseeable to access MAID if they suffer from a "grievous and irremediable medical condition" that "cannot be relieved under conditions that the patient considers acceptable." The new law also included a sunset provision, which after two years would expand the definition of "medical condition" to include a diagnosis of mental illness only. In addition, a recent government report recommended that lawmakers revisit the possibility of making MAID available to "mature minors." As we can see, the logical slippery slope argument is stronger than the typical slippery slope arguments that focus on the potential for abuse or neglect of safeguards, for it shows how regulations themselves are formed by precedent and practice.

There is a second, even more noteworthy, argument against PAS, one with a clearer connection to burdened agency. Advocates of PAS often make the distinction between the *offer of a choice*, which expands someone's freedom, and *coercion or manipulation*, which restricts freedom.[14] The assumption behind the distinction is that it can never be bad to increase someone's freedom by increasing her range of options. Whereas having fewer options may be harmful to us, having more options never can be.

David Velleman demonstrates, however, that it is not always better to have more options, for "having an option can be harmful even if we do not exercise it and—more surprisingly—even if we exercise it and gain by doing so."[15] It is not just that having to choose the nature and timing of your death (or the death of a loved one) is experienced as a burden. The more profound effect is that "having choices can . . . deprive one of desirable outcomes whose desirability depends on their being unchosen."[16] He gives the following example: "If I invite you to a dinner party, I leave you the possibilities of choosing to come or choosing to stay away; but I deprive you of something that you otherwise would have had—namely, the possibility of being absent from my table by default, as you are on all other evenings."[17] Placed in this situation, one's best option may be to accept the invitation and preserve the friendship. But one may do so lamenting the fact that one will no longer enjoy a relaxing night at home. According to Velleman, "these attitudes are consistent because refusing to attend a party is a different outcome from *not* attending without having to refuse."[18] In other words, "[one] can now choose the status quo or choose the alternative, but [one] can no longer *have* the status quo without *choosing* it."[19] The implications of this for vulnerable populations, including the elderly, are potentially troubling. As Banner points out, those who do not pursue PAS "will now be doing something they were previously not doing, namely *choosing not to die*. And in the way of such things, this 'choice' may come to stand in need of justification, and so admit of social criticism."[20] Thus, there enters in an added burden—the burden of having to justify one's continued existence!

If this conclusion seems far-fetched, consider Baroness Mary Warnock's controversial defense of the "duty to die." In a 2008 interview with the Scottish Presbyterian magazine *Life and Work*, she argued, "If you're demented, you're wasting people's lives—your family's lives—and you're wasting the resources of the National Health Service. . . . [In such cases] there's nothing wrong with feeling you ought to [die] for the sake of others as well as yourself."[21]

Hospice and palliative care, when considered in this light, fare much better. But these are no panaceas; they do not deliver anyone from the difficulties of burdened agency. For instance, the hospice philosophy of finding "personal meaning" in the dying process may be a popular concept in a pluralistic society such as our own. But if the institutions that provide the necessary framework for the construction of meaning are socially mediated, then we might reconsider any strategy that places the onus on the individual to construct his or her own meaning. As Daniel Callahan points out, "There can be nothing worse than concocted, self-conscious ritual, creating a make-believe world of sweetness and light to cover over the harshness of death. But serious customs and rituals, refined over time, can give a shape and context to grief and our understanding of death."[22]

Furthermore, neither of our current scripts are very applicable in the context of the most typical illness trajectories at the end of life (what researchers refer to as "prolonged dwindling"). Hospice is typically not medically indicated until one's life expectancy is less than six months. Because one might experience dwindling for up to ten years and because it can be difficult to determine when such decline has become "terminal," hospice is often not suggested until one is very close to actively dying. In 2014, for example, the average length of service was 71.3 days and the median (50th percentile) length of stay was 17.4 days, which means that about half of those who use hospice enter with fewer than 18 days of life remaining.[23]

PAS, at least under current regulations, requires a similar prognosis. For PAS, however, there is the added complication of determining patient competency. It is not uncommon during the course of prolonged dwindling to develop symptoms of dementia or mental illness (e.g., treatable depression). It is not clear that such patients are in a position to make a voluntary informed request for PAS. Indeed, the loss of capacity sometimes occurs before one can be given a terminal (<6 months) prognosis, making PAS an impossibility for many who would otherwise prefer it.

The concept of dwindling invites the question, when (along the prolonged course of life and eventual decline) can we begin to say of someone that he or she is "dying"? The answer, sadly, is often enough: when he or she is no longer economically productive—extracted from the labor force and demanding more resources than he or she is producing. The language associated with PAS and hospice sometimes falls into the trap of reinforcing the perpetuation of this economic logic as, for example, when each becomes a way to avoid "becoming a burden" on loved ones or society.

Nevertheless, despite all of these difficulties, many do turn to these scripts for dying. In the context of burdened agency, we either entrust our care to professionals who promise comfort and support in rejecting the technological "do-everything" approach to medicine or secure a "good death" by ending our life while our dignity, autonomy, and identity are still intact.

Many readers will find this all fairly unsurprising and straightforward; however, there is value in pressing a bit deeper precisely at the point where intuitions seem most self-explanatory and taken for granted. Why is it that certain goods or values (e.g., comfort, identity, autonomy, etc.) take on the particular importance for us that they do? In the language of philosopher Charles Taylor, why are these the "hypergoods . . . , [which] provide the standpoint from which [all other goods] must be weighed, judged, and decided about"?[24] To ask these sorts of questions of one's own culture can be a challenging task. And yet, it is a crucial one to which we will now turn.

MORAL AGENCY AND THE MODERN IDENTITY

Gnothi seauton—"Know thyself"—has long been considered the first task of gaining wisdom. Such knowledge is challenging enough on the individual level but is even more difficult for communities, people groups, and whole societies. Arguably, self-understanding is most difficult precisely where it seems least controversial—that is, where our intuitions seem to require no justification at all. To understand the background picture, or "social imaginary"[25] as Taylor calls it, lying behind our spiritual and moral intuitions involves bringing into focus not only how these intuitions come to expression in our communal and social practices but also a sense of the substantive beliefs about the world and human beings that underlie them.

In his profoundly influential book *Sources of the Self*, Taylor offers an account of "the modern identity," defined as "the ensemble of (largely unarticulated) understandings of what it is to be a human agent: the senses of inwardness, freedom, individuality, and being embedded in nature which are at home in the modern West."[26] Taylor's account illuminates why PAS and hospice have arisen as the most intuitive and visible responses to the crisis of technological brinkmanship and overly medicalized dying. According to Taylor, there are "three major facets" to the modern identity: a sense of inwardness, affirmation of ordinary life, and nature as a moral source. This section will offer a brief explanation of each and explain their significance for the rise of burdened agency and the turn toward our two scripts for dying.

Inwardness

The idea that we are such things as "selves" whose emotional, intellectual, and spiritual riches are the substance of our "inner lives," that we contain "inner depths" of being, and that the essential location of our selfhood is necessarily "within" us—these notions will strike many of us as so intuitively obvious that it might be difficult to accept Taylor's claims about their relative novelty. Although the roots of our notion of "inwardness" are very deep in our cultural history, its most fully developed version in which the sources of morality reside *within* us arose relatively recently. To be sure, there were precursors. Plato famously affirmed the primacy of reason over the passions, of the soul over the body, of contemplation over civic action. But Plato did "not use the inside/outside dichotomy to make his point,"[27] for his primary concern was highlighting a moral source that lies not within us but outside—namely, the forms that reason ought to discern and love.

A crucial step toward an inner-outer dichotomy, according to Taylor, came with Augustinian Christianity. Augustine "introduced the inwardness of radical reflexivity and bequeathed it to the Western tradition of thought."[28] For Augustine, "the road from the lower to the higher, the crucial shift in direction, passes through our attending to ourselves as *inner*." In Augustine's own words, "Do not go outward; return within yourself. In the inward man dwells truth."[29] After Augustine, it made sense to inquire about the state of one's "inner life" in a way that was rare before him. It is important to note, however, that "Augustine makes the step to inwardness . . . *because it is a step towards God*,"[30] who is *interior intimo meo et superior summo meo* (closer to me than I am to myself while infinitely above me). The Augustinian agent is defined by her dependence on God whose perfection goes far beyond her powers. This sense of creaturely dependence, though perhaps after Augustine more self-aware than ever before, relies on and acknowledges a moral source that transcends the self.

A series of Enlightenment thinkers would later initiate a more thorough-going transformation of our understanding of our moral sources by shifting them within individual moral agents. When Descartes set out to establish the indubitable foundations of philosophy, he eschewed dependence on tradition in favor of the famously individualistic and self-sufficient *cogito ergo sum*. Where Augustinian reflexivity—attention to self *as* moral or spiritual agent—aided in the development of *pietas*, the acknowledgment of one's dependence on God, Cartesian reflexivity is a crucial stage in the rejection and disparagement of such dependence. The human being has become both *homo faber* (man, the maker) and *homo ipse faber* (man, the self-maker).

This basic philosophical anthropology set forth by Descartes was taken up and expanded in distinct ways by John Locke and Immanuel Kant. Locke extended the notions of self-responsible freedom and independence from authority in the direction of a "punctual" self, understood in terms of immediate self-consciousness. This self, as a pure, independent consciousness not essentially related to past or future, continually maintains the capacity for radical "self-remaking."[31] Kant pressed the notion of self-responsible freedom and the internalization of moral sources even further by making rational autonomy the foundation of human dignity.

These strains, which Taylor traces from Plato and Augustine through Descartes, Locke, and Kant, contribute to our inescapable sense of interiority. The modern identity presupposes that selfhood is necessarily related to rationality, to self-responsible freedom, to self-consciousness, and to the capacities of self-making and self-remaking. When combined with nature as a moral source and the affirmation of ordinary life, they go a long way toward making sense of why particular scripts for dying make intuitive sense for us, even when these leave us feeling dissatisfied and ambivalent about their adequacy.

"Nature" as Moral Source

Since early in the modern period, the rationalist picture of the human being that finds its strongest expressions in Descartes, Locke, and Kant has been accompanied by another picture we might call "expressivist" or "Romantic." This stance is perhaps best exemplified by Michel de Montaigne. As his Enlightenment contemporaries were advocating a neo-stoic emphasis on rational self-control, Montaigne instead argued for the pursuit of self-knowledge and self-acceptance through the reappropriation of the "natural." Mastery over nature is not the goal so much as accommodation to it. This requires reflection on and recognition of appropriate limits. On this basis, Montaigne advocated (and, in his writings, exemplified) an intense practice of self-reflection. In Taylor's words, "the fight is in a sense to come to accept who we are."[32] "Who we are," however, is understood in an "intensely individual"[33] way. My answer to this question will not be (or should not be) the same as yours. Authenticity and the discovery of originality are the goals of self-reflection. Particularity, rather than universality, is the hallmark of the human identity.

For many thinkers in this Romantic tradition, to discover one's originality is to connect with "the inner élan, the voice or impulse"[34] of Nature (the capitalization is intentional). Consider, for example, William Wordsworth's poem "The Prelude."[35] In it, the poet casts the inner growth and development of his own spiritual and intellectual life into a modern epic on the scale of Milton's *Paradise Lost*. Wordsworth seeks to write "some philosophic song / of truth that cherishes our daily life, / with meditations passionate from deep / recesses in man's heart" (1.229–32). The themes of "affirmation of everyday life" (to be explored below) and "inner depths" converge in these lines. In plumbing the depths of his inner life, Wordsworth is driven to exalt "the prime and vital principle" in Nature:

> Here must thou be, O man,
> Strength to thyself—no helper hast thou here—
> Here keepest thou thy individual state:
> No other can divide with thee this work,
> No secondary hand can intervene
> To fashion this ability. 'Tis thine,
> The prime and vital principle is thine
> In the recesses of thy nature, far
> From any reach of outward fellowship,
> Else 'tis not thine at all.
> (13.188–97)

Wordsworth's poem is an extended reflection on Nature's ability to inspire and guide the human heart into an ever more responsive and authentic existence. At times resembling an ode to Nature, "The Prelude" extols a life open to the natural world: "I am content / with my own modest pleasure, and have lived / with God and Nature communing, removed / from little enmities and low desires" (2.428–31).

These rationalist and the expressivist traditions mutually reinforce our pervading sense of individualism but do so in radically different ways. In each tradition, we receive a different account of what constitutes "human dignity" and what role such dignity plays in our life projects and social ethics. In a rare moment of direct commentary on a contemporary social and political issue, Taylor elaborates the tension between these two stances in terms of their relevance to our ecological crisis. He may just as well be speaking about the difficulty we have of knowing how to exercise moral agency in dying:

> These two spiritual outlooks are in confrontation. One sees the dignity of man in his assuming control of an objectified universe through instrumental reason. . . . The other sees in this very stance to nature a purblind denial of our place in things. We ought to recognize that we are part of a larger order of living beings, in the sense that our life springs from there and is sustained from there. Recognizing this involves acknowledging a certain allegiance to this larger order . . . to take the argument in the reverse direction, taking up an instrumental stance is a denial of the need for this attunement. It is a kind of separation, a

statement a priori of our moral dependence, of our self-sufficiency. The battle between these spiritual outlooks, which starts in the eighteenth century, is still going on today.[36]

Is the ideal for moral agency to be found in the self-responsible task of bringing the contingencies of nature—including the fragility and vulnerability of our bodies to decay and death—under the influence of instrumental reason (the script of euthanasia)? Or is the moral ideal to be found in our attunement to the nature of embodiment as finite and mortal, in the correlative embrace of dependence and rejection of self-sufficiency (the script of hospice)? This basic tension underlies our public discourse about death and dying. There is, however, one additional element of the modern identity that must be brought into focus, which comes down to us filtered through both rationalist and the expressivist outlooks—namely, what Taylor calls the "affirmation of ordinary life."

Affirmation of Ordinary Life

The basic tension between control *of* nature and attunement *to* nature is overlaid with another feature of the modern identity: a strong affirmation of "ordinary life"—the life of labor, production, household management, marriage, and family. This is a stark contrast to the ancient classical hierarchy between the good life, understood as participation in a range of higher activities such as philosophical or spiritual contemplation, and a life consumed by the tasks necessary for the subsistence of merely biological life. Those with the means to be freed from "servile" responsibilities developed a life in pursuit of the "*liberal* arts" associated with philosophy, theology, and perhaps public service and politics.

The sense that the good life depends on freedom from the lower activities was carried forward from ancient classical ethics into the medieval monastic tradition until it was finally rejected by Martin Luther and the Protestant Reformers.[37] As is the case with other aspects of the modern identity, the impulse behind the affirmation of ordinary life was originally theological in nature.[38] As Max Weber once quipped, Luther abolished the monastery and made every man a monk. In the hands of the Reformers, "vocation" no longer referred to a special priestly calling but to the sphere of daily activity, be it farming, manufacturing and trade, homemaking, or governance. One important effect of this shift, as Weber pointed out, is the rise of the "Protestant work ethic," which, when paired with an ascetical morality, led to unprecedented gains in productivity, wealth, and capital accumulation.[39] A more important effect, however, at least for our purposes, is how the affirmation of ordinary life led to a related moral obligation that has become deeply intuitive for us—namely, the universal obligation to alleviate suffering.

One key episode in the development of this theme, briefly mentioned in the previous chapter, is the advent of Baconian science, which brought together an instrumental stance toward the world and the Puritan-inspired reform impulse. For Francis Bacon and his followers, the knowledge that is most important is knowledge that can be put to use in the service of universal human benevolence. "Knowledge is power," not only in the sense that knowledge makes us powerful but in the sense that what counts as knowledge is that which allows us to bring nature under our control for the welfare of humanity.

Under the influence of the Baconian worldview, "affirming ordinary life has meant valuing the efficacious control of things by which it is preserved and enhanced as well as valuing the detachment from purely personal enjoyments which would blunt our dedication to its general flourishing."[40] During the Enlightenment, in a manner that Taylor suggests was different from any time before, the moral ideals of universal benevolence and the affirmation of ordinary life converged to create a "moral imperative to reduce suffering.... We feel called on to relieve suffering, to put an end to it."[41] Of course, it would be folly to suggest that premodern people did not experience pity for the suffering of others or that they did not feel a deep aversion toward the suffering of neighbors and loved ones. What is important about the modern stance toward suffering is not the sense that it is to be avoided if possible but how intensely we feel our obligation to relieve suffering in virtually all forms regardless of the source or nature of such suffering or the identity of the suffering one. Not only are we much more sensitive to suffering but also different in the way we consider the obligation to reduce suffering at a minimum as part of what it means to respect the dignity of others.

CONCLUSION:
THE MODERN IDENTITY AND SCRIPTS FOR DYING

Taylor's account of the modern identity provides a valuable framework for understanding the conditions of burdened agency and why the two scripts of hospice and euthanasia hold such power today. When the avoidance of death and suffering takes on paramount importance, for example, every technological advantage must be employed in the fight against disease and death. The very availability of a potentially curative therapy or a means of life extension is considered self-justifying in such a way that makes it difficult not to use it. In the United States, the moral imperative to reduce suffering and the claims of equality and universal justice underlie our public programs like Medicare.

Medical anthropologist Sharon Kaufmann, for example, has argued that our sense of "ordinary medicine" is shaped by four major (but largely invisible) "health care drivers." These include (1) the biomedical research industry and the rapidly increasing number of clinical trials; (2) the committees that set the reimbursement and insurance payment policies at private insurance companies but especially at Medicare; (3) the fact that a Medicare-reimbursable technology is almost instantly established as "standard of care"; and (4) the fact that "standard" therapies are considered "ethically necessary and therefore difficult, if not impossible, for physicians, patients and families to refuse."[42] Kaufmann emphasizes the moral presuppositions behind the formation of Medicare:

> The two ethical decisions undergirding the Medicare program, which came into being in 1965, were, first, that "it was incumbent on government to guarantee health care for the elderly," and second, that the cost of drugs, devices, procedures, and all treatments would not determine how, when, and how much technology was used. In the industrialized world this ethical decision—to provide government payment for medical care to the elderly (and for the poor through Medicaid) with no cost limitation—was and remains unique in that if a treatment is deemed useful, Medicare has a *moral imperative* to pay for it. That mandate is the core value of the Medicare program.[43]

The way Medicare decisions are made and the factors that are allowed to play into such decisions are informed by basic notions of justice, equality, and universal benevolence. Unfortunately, an unintended consequence has been the tendency to utilize every available means in the fight against death and suffering, often leading to overtreatment and undesirable forms of dying, as we have already noted at length. The response of the medical establishment to this conundrum has largely been to emphasize individual rights and patient autonomy. While this may be an improvement over paternalistic medicine, it also contributes to burdened agency. Indeed, it merely shifts the burden from the physician to the patient.

PAS and (voluntary) euthanasia represent the next step on the trajectory, which brings together strong emphasis on avoidance of suffering and the individual's autonomy rights. Perhaps nowhere in our culture are the two brought so closely together. The language of "compassion" predominates the discourse around PAS, but the assumption that PAS is primarily motivated by a desire to avoid a painful death is misleading. As much of the "right to die" rhetoric reveals, the most fundamental issue for advocates of PAS is maintaining control. To be sure, many of the advocates are also motivated by a desire to ease suffering at the end of life, but the fact is that pain and fear of pain are not primary motivations for those who request PAS.[44] The most relevant aspect of the suffering that the "death with dignity" movement seeks to prevent is the loss of a certain sort of rational agency and the dissolution of personal identity.

But the loss of rational agency does not necessarily entail a threat to dignity. It is, of course, possible to see human rationality as a valuable trait, while holding open the possibility for other sources of human dignity.[45] In the modern identity, however, rational freedom has become something more than a mere occasion for respect; it is (especially in its Kantian formulation) the loadstone of our moral sources. Apart from the concepts of self-responsible freedom or rational autonomy, we struggle to imagine any notion of what the good life could entail or how we could muster the inspiration necessary to attain it.

As we have seen, this account of dignity is not the only one that is present in our culture. Expressivist notions about the value of individuality, particularity, and authenticity give rise to an understanding that locates human dignity in the depths of nature or in the creative imagination. Hospice and palliative care tend to embrace and draw on this second strand. While pain is managed, drugs are generally limited as much as possible to give people every opportunity to work through the "personal meaning" of their journey toward death. Hospice caretakers are increasingly focusing on the development of a "personal narrative" as a way of helping patients find meaning at the end of life.[46] Sociologist Tony Walter claims that dying today "is essentially personal. Its hallmarks are choice and personal expression."[47] The central authority figure is no longer the priest or the doctor but the self. The dominant discourse is no longer theology or medicine but psychology. In its emphasis on personal meaning, forged by the recognition of (and attunement to) finitude and limitation, hospice indeed taps into this expressivist notion of human identity and human dignity.

A final note: Although presented as competing scripts, hospice and euthanasia actually share certain fundamental characteristics including a critique of medicalized dying and a desire to avoid death in the ICU. But there is a second commonality; according to Michael Banner, "both movements are . . . imbued with notions central to projects of self-expression and preservation of identity, characteristic of late modernity."[48] The goal of preserving agency and individuality is shared, but the strategies diverge: "Hospice care bids to preserve and maintain the project of the self for as long as possible up until the occurrence of biological death; euthanasia brings death forwards so as to avoid the risk of the death of the self prior to biological death."[49] The effects of this commonality on the burdened agent are ambivalent. On the one hand, this emphasis on agency and individuality may be a necessary first step toward finding innovative modalities of dying that ease the strain. On the other hand, this merely reinforces the cultural dynamics that fuel burdened agency in the first place. Neither script delivers us from the perplexities of choice in dying and the sense that we are ill-equipped to manage the responsibility we bear.

Burdened agency is reinforced by a complex web of assumptions that permeate the modern social imaginary—assumptions about personhood and agency, about dignity and control, about identity and authenticity, and about suffering and meaning. The relationship between this web of assumptions and specifically Christian notions of humanity, meaning, and identity is a complicated one. Many of the features of our social imaginary are rooted in Christian theological notions—transformed, to be sure, into a largely secular framework and narrative. Nevertheless, in the following chapters, I will argue that Christian understandings of theological anthropology and human agency, especially in relation to death and dying, subvert many of the fundamental cultural assumptions outlined in the previous two chapters. In its discerning how to relate to the fact of human mortality—and to our own particular deaths—Christianity has articulated forms of agency that are not entirely consonant with certain assumptions of modernity.

THREE

Persons, Freedom, and a Catholic Spirituality of Martyrdom

DEATH AND DYING IN THE ROMAN CATHOLIC TRADITION

Philosopher Margaret Battin has suggested that we live amid a great divide between "Stoic" and "Christian" approaches to death and dying. Culturally, we are of two minds about "the individual's role in his or her own death: whether one's role should be as far as possible active, self-assertive, and responsible and may include ending one's own life—or, on the other hand, acceptant, obedient, and passive in the sense of being patient, where 'allowing to die' is the most active step that should be taken."[1] Battin's dichotomy contrasts responsibility with patience and obedience. It also contrasts activity with passivity. In both cases, Christianity is identified with the latter but not the former.

But is this really a fair way of describing the Christian perspective on agency in dying? As is often the case in such matters, things are more complex than this dichotomy suggests. "Active" and "passive" do not capture the subtle forms of agency available through Christian theological sources. Furthermore, patience and obedience are often appropriate ways of being properly responsible. In what follows, I explain how Roman Catholic moral theology provides a rich and profound body of reflection on death and dying that yields a more textured account of human agency in dying than Battin's dichotomy suggests. The *Catechism of the Catholic Church* provides the basic contours of the traditional Christian doctrines on death and dying, so I will begin with an overview of its teachings.[2] Two prominent Jesuit theologians then represent different ways of developing the Catholic perspective. Richard McCormick, S.J., gives a personalist natural-law approach that highlights the relationship between decision making at the end of life and the various goods of a human life considered as a whole. Karl Rahner, S.J., offers a Christian existentialist understanding of death as a personal act and opportunity to demonstrate faithful surrender before the divine. A Catholic approach to agency in dying, I argue, is best summed up in Servais Pinckaers, O.P.'s, notion of a "spirituality of martyrdom," which understands the goal of the Christian moral life as faithful witness to the point of death. This Catholic theological approach reveals deep flaws in a simple active-passive binary understanding of agency in dying, and rejects the assumption that freedom and responsibility requires setting aside obedience and patience. It also places attention on the process of spiritual formation that occurs throughout one's life, which ultimately affects one's experience of agency at the end of life. The spirituality of martyrdom, as I will develop it, has the potential to engender a new vision of the dying process that provides an alternative to the modern social imaginary which has perpetuated the problems of burdened agency.

The *Catechism*'s Teachings on Death

The *Catechism of the Catholic Church* (hereafter CCC) teaches that the first human pair initially enjoyed perfect fellowship and harmony with God that permeated all aspects of their life and preserved them in a state of "original justice." In this state, human beings were "mortal" but were not "destined to die" (CCC, 1.2.3.11.2). "As long as he remained in the divine intimacy, man would not have to suffer or die" (CCC, 1.2.1.1.6). The prohibition against eating from the "'tree of the knowledge of good and evil' symbolically evokes the insurmountable limits that man, being a creature, must freely recognize and respect with trust" (CCC, 1.2.1.1.7). In choosing to eat of this tree, the human being "chose himself over God" and attempted to be like God (*sicut Deus*) "without God, before God, and not in accordance with God" (CCC, 1.2.1.1.7). This choice had the momentous repercussion of dissolving the state of original justice and disrupting the harmony between the soul and body, eventuating in the dissolution and destruction of their unity in death. In this way, "death makes its entrance into human history" (CCC, 1.2.1.1.7).

Notably, under this conception, human death enters God's creation as a result of human action, and both action and result run counter to God's original intention for human beings (CCC, 1.2.3.11.2). For support of this position, the *Catechism* cites the Book of Wisdom (1:13, 2:24): "God did not make death, and he does not delight in the death of the living. . . . It was through the devil's envy that death entered the world." Nevertheless, human beings are not understood to have been created with natural immortality. In Thomas Aquinas's words, death is "in one way natural, in another unnatural." Before the fall, "the human body was not indissoluble by reason of any intrinsic vigor of immortality, but by reason of a supernatural force given by God to the soul, whereby it was enabled to preserve the body from all corruption so long as it remained itself subject to God. . . . This favor was withdrawn due to the sin of the first parents. Accordingly, death is both natural on account of a condition attaching to matter, and a punishment on account of the loss of the Divine gift preserving the human being from death."[3] On this view, God does not alter human nature by *making* human beings mortal but rather allows the natural course of death to occur. Nevertheless, when death occurs, it is "unnatural," for it leads to separation of the soul from the body, leaving each alienated from its telos, or perfection.[4]

The *Catechism* returns to the theme of human mortality when it presents the Church's teaching on the death of Christ. In his crucifixion and burial, Jesus did not only "die for our sins" but also "tasted death," experiencing the condition of the separation of body and soul. On Holy Saturday, Christ "descended into hell" to save the righteous ones (including Adam and Eve) who had gone before him. Interestingly, the tradition seems to hedge a bit at this point, stressing that Jesus's death was a "real death" (i.e., separation of body and soul) but adds that his body retained a union with the person of the Son, so that "his was not a mortal corpse like others" and did not experience decay (CCC, 1.2.2.4.3).

Pastoral and Ethical Guidance on Dying

The *Catechism* goes beyond laying out the doctrinal basics for a general understanding of death and mortality and addresses dying as a moral issue for the Christian. How is the believer to understand and approach her death? She is first to recognize that bodily death is "in a sense . . . natural." The awareness of the fact that like all living things, we will develop, grow old, and eventually die should lend a sense of urgency to our lives: remembering our mortality helps us realize that we have only a limited time in which to bring our lives to fulfillment (CCC, 1.2.2.5.1; cf. Eccles 12:1). Death is the end of one's earthly pilgrimage, closing the period during which one works out one's eternal destiny (Heb 9:27). Even though "death seems like the normal end of life," however, the magisterium is also clear that it is in fact "the wages of sin," contrary to the plan of God, and "the last enemy" to be destroyed. It is not, in and of itself, a good or natural thing.

There is room, however, for a legitimate "experience of a desire for death" (CCC, 1.2.2.5.1). This is possible because Jesus, through his free obedience and submission unto death, has "transformed the curse of death into a blessing." If the believer, through the sacrament of baptism, has already been incorporated into Christ's death and resurrection, then physical death becomes the completion of this incorporation and a "passing over" into the presence of God. The *Catechism* sees "dying in Christ" as the ultimate fulfillment of the entire Christian sacramental life: "For the Christian the day of death inaugurates, at the end of his sacramental life, the fulfillment of his new birth begun at Baptism, the definitive 'conformity' to 'the image of the Son' conferred by the anointing of the Holy Spirit, and participation in the feast of the Kingdom which was anticipated in the Eucharist—even if final purifications are still necessary for him in order to be clothed with the nuptial garment" (CCC, 2.2.4.2.1).

On the traditional view, death is an evil, though not the greatest evil, and life is a good, though not the greatest good.[5] If, then, death can be legitimately desired by the Christian, can it be intentionally sought and brought about? Here, the magisterium answers clearly in the negative. On the topic of suicide, the *Catechism* stresses that life is a gift that comes from God but in such a way that God "remains sovereign Master of life" (CCC, 3.2.2.5.1).[6] In light of that fact, each person is "responsible for his life" and should "accept [it] gratefully and preserve it," remembering that each of us is a "steward, not owner, of the life God has entrusted us" (CCC, 3.2.2.5.1). The *Catechism* provides several specific reasons why suicide is considered a serious moral offence, including (a) as mentioned, it places the human being unjustly in the place of God as the one with proper authority to dispose of life; (b) the act of suicide runs counter to the natural and proper desire for self-preservation; (c) it violates self-love; (d) it violates neighbor love by breaking one's ties of solidarity with one's family and community; and (e) it runs counter to the love of God by failing to accept the gift of life appropriately. Although the *Catechism* urges an agnostic, yet hopeful, stance regarding the possibility of the eternal salvation of those who take their own lives and although it acknowledges circumstances that may mitigate the guilt incurred in such an act, it nevertheless holds that any act of intentional self-killing is a violation of the law of God as expressed in the fifth commandment.[7]

For similar reasons, the magisterium likewise condemns medical assistance in dying, as well as acts of euthanasia, as morally unacceptable.[8] Any "act or omission which, of itself or by intention, causes death in order to eliminate suffering constitutes a murder gravely contrary to the dignity of the human person and to the respect due to the living God, his Creator" (CCC, 3.2.2.5.1). This holds true no matter what motive lies behind the act (e.g., a compassionate desire to relieve suffering) or what means is used to carry it through. For instance, the *Catechism* explicitly forbids the interruption of "ordinary care," like artificial nutrition and hydration, "even if death is thought imminent" (CCC, 3.2.2.5.1).[9]

The magisterium draws a distinction between passive euthanasia and the withdrawal or withholding of treatments that are considered "burdensome, dangerous, extraordinary, disproportionate . . . [or] 'over-zealous'" (CCC, 3.2.2.5.1). Such procedures may be legitimately refused even if doing so will knowingly lead to death which may otherwise have been delayed. Although the magisterium rejects ending life to alleviate suffering, it does not reject the desire to alleviate suffering. Palliative care is upheld as a proper aim of medicine: it is good and right to relieve suffering when possible. Suffering, however, is not treated as an inherently "meaningless" phenomenon but rather may be "an opportunity for sharing in a particular way in the Lord's Cross, the source of spiritual fruitfulness."[10] Furthermore, the magisterium allows for the use of medicine to alleviate suffering, even at the risk of hastening death, so long as "death is not willed as either an end or a means, but only foreseen and tolerated as inevitable" (CCC, 3.2.2.5.1). The underlying principle given: "Here one does not will to cause death; [rather] one's inability to impede it is merely accepted" (CCC, 3.2.2.5.1). As one commentator sums up the moral stance of the Roman Catholic magisterium, "The Christian should neither exhaust life to avoid death nor administer death before the Author of life."[11]

Some Preliminary Observations

At this point, note the following about the teaching of the magisterium. (1) For Catholicism, the basic unit of moral analysis has generally been the discrete *act*. Morality concerns human acts, which are understood to be free exercises of intellect and volition.[12] In this tradition, to determine the *rightness or wrongness* of an act (i.e., its moral "*species*"), one must first answer the question, what is being done? This process, called specification, involves determining the moral object of the act in question. The "object" is "the proximate end of a deliberate decision," that at which it aims. Such an end may be distinguished from the agent's subjective desire or motivation.[13] The moral object names the objective, or intrinsic, end of an action — the "end" determined not by the subjective experience of the actor but by the very nature of the act. Roman Catholic moral theology holds certain acts to be intrinsically and inescapably wrong by virtue of their moral object.[14] Following the Pauline principle that a good end may not be pursued by an evil means (Rom 3:8), the magisterium holds that an act whose object is wrong or evil cannot be made right or good by virtue of a benevolent motivation.[15] Euthanasia, suicide, physician-assisted suicide (PAS), and withdrawal of artificial nutrition and hydration (AN&H), according to the magisterium, are all considered "intrinsically evil" because they are intrinsically ordered toward bringing about a person's death. They, therefore, offend against "the incomparable and inviolable worth of every human life."[16]

(2) Although the magisterium strictly forbids acts that aim directly at death, it does allow for, and even endorses, the use of medications to relieve suffering and pain. It even allows for "terminal sedation," which involves the administration of narcotic drugs that relieve pain and suffering, while also reducing consciousness and hastening death.[17] Here, the tradition relies on the rule of double effect, which states that a person may morally act in a way that brings about an evil effect (in this case, death), so long as (a) that person does not directly intend the evil effect, (b) the person intends and brings about a good effect that is proportional to the evil effect, (c) the act is not "intrinsically evil," and (d) the evil effect is not itself the means by which the good effect is secured.

The case of "terminal sedation" simultaneously illustrates the usefulness of double-effect reasoning and its limitations. Those who care for patients at the end of life know firsthand the relief that such drugs may bring in a person's final hours. Many, however, believe deeply in the importance of the Hippocratic maxim, "First, do no harm," and its expression (in the modern Oath) in the refusal to administer deadly "poisons" to any person— presumably even for humanitarian purposes. For such people, the principle of double effect allows them to affirm both truths at once. Many will admit, however, that given the close proximity between administering such palliative measures and the advent of death, it is not always quite so clear that death is not, in fact, "intended." Although this has caused many to question and even reject the principle of double effect,[18] the magisterium nevertheless uses such logic to affirm the legitimacy of terminal sedation (though, notably, it does caution that terminal sedation removes the patient from the dying role and therefore should be avoided, if possible, so that she may prepare "herself with full consciousness for meeting Christ").[19]

(3) Finally, the magisterium employs a distinction between "ordinary" (or "proportionate") medical care, on the one hand, and "extraordinary" (or "disproportionate") medical care, on the other hand. According to the United States Conference of Catholic Bishops, "proportionate means [of preserving life] are those that in the judgment of the patient offer a reasonable hope of benefit and do not entail an excessive burden, or impose excessive expense on the family or community."[20] If such means exist, according to the magisterium, they are considered obligatory. "Extraordinary" or "disproportionate" means, however, are never required of patients and

physicians in the pursuit of health or life. According to the Congregation for the Doctrine of Faith (CDF), when death is imminent, it is not a rejection of life to reject treatments that "would only secure a precarious and burdensome prolongation of life, so long as the normal care due to the sick person in similar cases is not interrupted."[21] As we will see momentarily, such terms as "burdensome prolongation of life" and "normal care" are open to considerably wide interpretation.

RICHARD MCCORMICK'S REVISIONIST NATURAL-LAW APPROACH

Assessing Quality of Life?

Richard McCormick's work in practical ethics and moral theology brings to the fore additional complexities in the Catholic approach to moral agency at the end of life. While at times pressing up against the magisterium's teaching, that he did not fully embrace something like PAS shows that he remained committed to a view of human agency in dying that is in line with the Catholic teachings.

In an early article, McCormick engaged nascent debates about the ethics of withdrawing life-sustaining medical interventions from critically ill newborns. In it, he describes a medical case involving a premature newborn with multiple complications, including major deformities of ear, eye, hand, vertebrae, and esophagus. The child quickly contracted pneumonia and, because of poor circulation, almost certainly had severe brain damage. The parents declined consent for physicians to perform reparative surgery on the child's tracheal esophageal fistula, sparking an appeal by the physicians to the Maine superior court. The judge ruled in favor of the physicians and against the parents, citing the child's inalienable right to life.

The conclusion of the court, McCormick notes, though true in the strictest sense, nevertheless failed to address the deeper issue of whether a considerably dubious prognosis might call into question the conclusion that a "right to life" necessarily entails a duty to extend that life. For example, it seems unreasonable to assume that the life of an anencephalic newborn must in every case be indefinitely prolonged by mechanical and artificial means. Of course, there is a very real danger on the other side as well. Consider the (in)famous "Johns Hopkins case," which involved an infant with Down syndrome and duodenal atresia (i.e., intestinal obstruction). In this case, the parents refused consent for a fairly simple procedure to remedy the obstruction, resulting in the child's death by starvation after fifteen days in the hospital. McCormick observes that such a case is morally indefensible. Taking these cases together highlights the importance of the following series of questions: "Which infants, if any, should be allowed to die? On what grounds or according to what criteria, as determined by whom?"[22] Is it possible to push past slogans (like "Death with dignity" or "Right to life") and articulate some substantial ethical standards for guiding the decision-making process in such cases?

As noted, historically the distinction between "ordinary" and "extraordinary means" guided deliberation about withholding and withdrawing life-prolonging medical treatment. According to the American Medical Association (at the time of McCormick's writing), "the cessation of the employment of extraordinary means to prolong the life of the body when there is irrefutable evidence that biological death is imminent is the decision of the patient and/or his immediate family." With the development of many lifesaving and life-prolonging technologies, however, the issue of withholding and withdrawing possible treatments no longer hinges on being able to say that biological death is "imminent" for a patient. After all, "contemporary medicine," notes McCormick, "can keep almost anyone alive."[23] The case of neonates with multiple life-threatening complications makes this dynamic especially acute. In such cases, "the questions, 'Is this means too hazardous or difficult to use?' and 'Does this measure only prolong the patient's dying?' while still useful and valid, now often become, 'Granted that we can easily save the life, what kind of life are we saving?' This is a quality-of-life judgment. And we fear it."[24] This puts caregivers in a "position of awesome responsibility"[25] that comes along with burdened agency.

A Personalist Approach to End-of-Life Decisions

Just because it is possible to extend mere life practically indefinitely does not mean that is always the right thing to do. We need some sort of principles to discern when it is and when it is not. But we also must be careful lest these decisions hinge on "quality of life" judgments that merely reinforce the prejudices of the one making the assessment. In 1957, Pope Pius XII spoke to a group of physicians about end-of-life medical decisions. According to the pope, a treatment is considered *extraordinary* if it is "too burdensome for most men and would render the attainment of the higher, more important good too difficult. Life, death, all temporal activities are in fact *subordinate* to spiritual ends."[26] This statement confirms, for McCormick, that Catholic morality treats life as a basic and precious but relative good. Biological life is not simply an end in itself but rather is "a good to be preserved precisely as the condition of other values."[27] McCormick identifies these "higher goods" as the love of God and of neighbor—"the meaning, substance, and consummation of life are found in human *relationships*, and . . . the qualities of justice, respect, concern, compassion, and support that surround them."[28] Where the "importance of relationships gets lost in the struggle for survival," we should suspect that something has gone wrong. "It is neither inhuman nor un-Christian to say that there comes a point where an individual's condition itself represents the negation of any truly human—that is, relational—potential."[29]

Placing relational potential at the center of quality of life reflects McCormick's deep commitment to "personalism," a theological and moral vision of "free, creative, and acting persons engaged in an adventure of responsible liberty in which people unite with others to create a society in which the structures, customs, and institutions both shape and are shaped by the nature of the person."[30] McCormick considered the Church's articulation of "integral personalism" to be a "conciliar achievement" of Vatican II, in full display in documents like *Gaudium et Spes*.[31] Drawing on the "principle of totality,"[32] *Gaudium et Spes* (#51) asserted that the "moral aspect of any [medical] procedure . . . must be determined by objective standards which are based on the nature of the person and the person's acts." McCormick observes that the official commentary indicates that the choice of this wording means that "human activity must be judged insofar as it refers to the human person integrally and adequately considered (*personam humanam integre et adequate considerandum*)." McCormick takes this to mean that all aspects or dimensions of human personhood—including personal subjectivity, responsible freedom, and relationality (which includes attention to the communities and institutions around the person)—are relevant for evaluating a moral act.

The effect of McCormick's personalism is to widen the range of relevant factors necessary for morally evaluating acts that hasten death. McCormick is not interested in an evaluation of one's subjective experience along utilitarian lines, as if to calculate the expected marginal utility (the balance of pleasure over pain) over the course of one's remaining life. The presence of even a fairly diminished form of relational capacity would suffice, in McCormick's view, to justify measures to secure and protect an endangered life, even in the face of certain hardships. McCormick repeatedly emphasizes the inevitability of human suffering and its potential to become meaningful. With respect to the issue of withholding and withdrawing treatment, however, McCormick's central claim is that "the very purpose of life can be put at risk by serious illness and physical suffering even more than by death" itself.[33] When the efforts to sustain life impede the attainment of the higher goods embodied in Jesus's love command (Mark 12:28–31; John 13:34) or do not stand a reasonable chance at enabling such goods, it may be acceptable to forgo them.

It is worth noting that McCormick cites an additional reason for emphasizing the centrality of the person ("integrally and adequately understood")—namely, in so doing, "it becomes clear that a moral assessment of our actions must consider the *whole action*—external act, intention, circumstances, consequences—for each of its aspects has an effect upon the person."[34] Thus, for McCormick, an acceptance of personalism leads intrinsically and naturally to a more capacious analysis of human actions. This led many to associate him with "proportionalism," a position that has been opposed by both the magisterium and prominent natural-law philosophers who desire to uphold the legitimacy of moral absolutes against acts understood as "intrinsically" wrong or evil.[35] Critics of proportionalism assert that it amounts to a veiled form of consequentialism.

The key question is this: what is to count as pertaining to the moral object and moral species of an act? The *Catechism of the Catholic Church* defines the moral object as "a good toward which the will deliberately directs itself." This definition refers to the objective, or intrinsic, end of an action—the "end" determined not by the subject's motivation but by the very nature of the act itself. In other words, *what is it that is being done?* Moral species refers to the kind of action it is, whether it is right or wrong (or neutral). James Childress notes, "Proportionalists insist that moral species terms, which identify the moral nature of acts, do include or should include more than the mere physical, material event; they do or should include the whole set of morally relevant circumstances, as the prohibition of murder does but the prohibition of [killing] does not. Only where these circumstances are included can a prohibition be considered absolute."[36]

We don't know if a particular act of killing is an instance of murder unless we first know whether the act was, for example, unjust or justified, direct or indirect, intentional or unintended, whether the victim was innocent or deserving of death, and whether the agent was acting privately or in a position of legitimate authority. As this example demonstrates, to say that an act of murder is morally evil *ex objecto* (from its object) is *already* to account for a series of characteristics that exclude the possibility of moral exceptions. Proportionalists like McCormick do not object to absolute moral prohibitions; they simply insist that a similar process of specification occurs for all acts that are "intrinsically evil" and a priori morally wrong.

McCormick on Euthanasia and PAS

One might think that proportionalism would lead to a ready acceptance of PAS, but that was not the case for McCormick. Lisa Cahill notes, "McCormick was never willing to say that life could be taken directly to protect the moral integrity or dignity of the person. His analytical framework and vocabulary might have suggested a different outcome."[37] McCormick never openly disagreed with the magisterial teaching on euthanasia, and it is not clear that the teaching about AN&H that he did oppose was universally binding at the time.

Why did McCormick hesitate here? Cahill believes this was a matter of "prudence," a recognition of the dangers and potential risks of wide social acceptance of mercy killing. His resistance was not specifically related to the "intrinsic morality of individual acts" but "the possible short- and long-term effects of accepting acts of commission that result in death."[38] Perhaps this is true. There are certainly places where McCormick seems to take such a pragmatic line of approach.[39] He is clearly concerned with the negative effects of broader social attitudes toward death on our ability to make wise moral decisions in this sphere, insisting at one point that "until our culture has a healthy Christian attitude toward death, it cannot trust the answers it gives and must give to the many extremely difficult questions involved in any acceptance of positive euthanasia."[40] This is not exactly an overt rejection of euthanasia.

Does McCormick leave open the door to a general acceptance of euthanasia? Would adopting a more Christian attitude toward death lead to a more tolerant stance on mercy killing? McCormick does not say. In a discussion of Paul Ramsey, he seems to accept that there are instances in which the patient is "irretrievably inaccessible to human care." In such cases, the duty to care is no longer binding, for no one is bound to do the impossible. If this is true, then "the difference between omission and commission would seem to lose moral meaning; for the stricture against commission (positively causing death) is but a negative concretization of our duty to care."[41] McCormick, however, is quite cautious about accepting this line of thought, citing the dubious nature of judgments that classify patients in this way. Notably, his reasons for hesitating do not hinge on a rule-utilitarian type of argument. And this is why Cahill's conclusion may be slightly misguided, for it seems to add grist to the mill for those who want to charge McCormick with abandoning the deontology of natural law and absolute moral norms in favor of a consequentialist form of moral reasoning, albeit perhaps of a "refined" sort.[42]

McCormick's reluctance to embrace active euthanasia was in fact driven by core theological convictions.[43] According to McCormick, the death and resurrection of Christ radically reorients our disposition and attitude toward dependence. Our culture tends to see dependence on others as a terrible and terribly undignified fate, but "Christ's supreme dignity *was manifest* in dependence."[44] McCormick suggests that Christians should therefore embrace a theology of dependence: "Dependence on others should be a sign of our more radical dependence on God. Since our freedom is intended to lead us into a deeper union with God, it is an interesting paradox that our deep dependence on God establishes our own radical independence: independence in dependence."[45] In other words, we are *freed* from our compulsive need to be in-dependent.

McCormick extends these themes in his most explicit statement on euthanasia and PAS. In this article, McCormick contends that the absolutization of autonomy leads to "an intolerance of dependence on others." As a result, "Death with Dignity" has been reduced to dying "in *my way*, at *my time*, by *my hand*."⁴⁶ But this neglects the many ways in which human relationships depend on a dynamic of giving and taking. In other words, interdependence includes both independence and dependence—without each, we risk distorting the very meaning of human life.

Ultimately, the reason that McCormick rejects PAS (and, by extension, euthanasia) is that it represents not a compassionate response to an intractable and devastating problem but rather a symptom of (a) our unwillingness to deal with the distortions of care that make PAS seem desirable (e.g., inadequate pain management, the financial pressures of health care, the frequency of pointless and inhumane prolongation of the dying process, etc.) and (b) our reluctance to cultivate an acceptance of the place of limits and dependence in the context of the truly human life. Where one might expect proportionalism to aid in the acceptance of euthanasia, we see instead a theologically rich personalism preventing such a conclusion. Indeed, with McCormick, we see how core theological convictions supply resources for an alternative view of human agency (agency in dependence), thereby subverting the social imaginary that makes PAS and euthanasia seem like legitimate options.

KARL RAHNER'S *THEOLOGY OF DEATH*

Death as a Natural End

A similar notion of human agency is present in the more theologically substantive work of Karl Rahner. In his book *Zur Theologie des Todes* (On the theology of death), Rahner considers death under three aspects: (a) death as an event concerning the human being as a whole, (b) death as the consequence of sin, and (c) death as a dying with Christ—with an additional epilogue on the meaning and significance of Christian martyrdom.⁴⁷

Central to Rahner's theology of death is a basic tenet: The human being is a union of nature and person. The natural aspect of the human condition includes the limitations of organic, bodily life, subject to physical laws (e.g., the second law of thermodynamics, the necessity of sleep and consuming organic life for sustenance, etc.). In addition to the natural, human existence is also personal, characterized chiefly by freedom and self-determination. Personal life has a moral and spiritual dimension not captured in terms of human nature. The personal and the natural, however, are equiprimordial, we might say: the human being lives in a basic dialectical tension between freedom and finitude.[48]

According to Rahner, "death is an event which strikes man in his totality" (13). It must, then, have both a natural and a personal dimension. Rahner makes two main points about death's natural aspect. First, Rahner notes that natural death is universal. This statement goes beyond the purely empirical observation that all human beings die; it is about "more than an obscure, unsolved, purely biological problem" (14). Rahner notes, what is still the case today, that it remains a mystery "why all living things composed of many cells, and man in particular, do die" (15).[49] Nevertheless, Rahner (presciently) rejects the idea that death could, in principle, be removed from the human condition: "the necessity of death belongs to the necessary features of human existence. . . . It will never be possible to abolish death" (15). The second point Rahner makes about the natural aspect of death is that death is understood properly as the separation of body and soul. That this describes death as natural rather than personal may strike some as counterintuitive. Rahner himself notes that this classical theological formulation is "closer to the essence of death," but it still considers death naturally, for it approaches death from the point of view of the human being as organism. At death, "the soul no longer holds the structure of the body together as a distinct reality, governed by its own immanent, vital laws" (17).

"Separated" turns out to be a key word for Rahner's analysis. The teaching of the Church is that the soul does not cease to exist at death. But what relationship the soul retains, if any, to the material world remains unspecified. Rahner posits that since the soul is united with the body in life, it has an intrinsic relationship with the whole of which the body is a part—that is, the material cosmos. Rahner rejects the idea that at death, the soul's relation to the world is dissolved completely. The soul becomes not a-cosmic (a more Neoplatonic ideal than Christian) but rather more like "all-cosmic," entering into a "deeper, more comprehensive openness" toward the "ground of the unity of the universe" (19). Rahner is careful to note that this does not mean that the entire world becomes the "body" of the soul or that the soul becomes "omnipresent" (20–22). Rather, Rahner has in mind a more open and fluid relationship, a mysterious interpenetration, between soul and world, whereby the soul "becomes open towards the universe and, in some way, a co-determining factor of the universe" (22).

Death as Personal Act

The universality of death and the separation of body and soul are natural aspects of death that apply equally to all human beings. There is, however, a further, personal aspect of death: it is the conclusion of one's state of spiritual pilgrimage. As such, it "brings man, as a moral and spiritual person, a kind of finality and consummation which renders his decision for or against God, reached during the time of his bodily life, final and unalterable" (26). Behind this view of death as a personal act of fulfillment lies Rahner's understanding of the nature of human freedom and the "fundamental option." The relationship between the two is nicely summed up by Shannon Craigo-Snell: "Freedom, for Rahner, is not a neutral capacity to choose between options in a stream of individual choices. Rather, it is the freedom to decide about oneself in one's totality and in relation to God. It is the freedom to accept or reject one's orientation to God. . . . This choice, or fundamental option, is granted eternal validity by God."[50]

In the phrase "freedom to decide about oneself in one's totality," we see the influence of one of Rahner's teachers, Martin Heidegger. One of the central questions in Heidegger's *Being and Time* is how one is able to achieve "authenticity" in one's life. For Heidegger, the human mode of being (Dasein) is unique in that it considers the Being (i.e., the essential nature) of beings—including its own Being. In doing so, it recognizes Being as both meaningful and contingent, confronting Dasein with unrealized potentialities that provide possible ways forward. Dasein does not develop as an acorn develops into a tree. "Uniquely among beings, Dasein's existence precedes and determines its essence. Thus, Dasein's existence manifests what Heidegger calls 'mineness.'"[51] This opens up the possibility for genuinely free responsibility but also the possibility for its opposite: the refusal of responsible, individual agency in the world. The default state of Dasein, on Heidegger's view, is one in which individual responsibility is wrapped up in impersonal conventions about "what is [typically] done." Individuality—one's ownmost existence—is forfeited for inauthenticity, a mode of being that Heidegger calls "falling."

Death plays a central role in Dasein's achievement of true authenticity. Death's importance, for Heidegger, does not simply lie at the singular event that occurs at the end of biological life but also in one's existential attitude toward that event.[52] To be human is to be aware, deep down, of one's thrown-ness (*Geworfenheit*) toward death. In light of this awareness, one must determine how to relate to one's finite condition. Death does not remain a bare fact, but it becomes a *possibility*. This illuminates one's entire orientation toward the future as also "possibility" (*Möglichkeit*). Will the individual take responsibility for her future possibilities and especially for this "ownmost, nonrelational, certain, and, as such, indefinite and insuperable possibility" (i.e., death)?[53] If she will, Matthias Remenyi notes, "death loses its imposing aspect that plunges the subject into radical passivity . . . and becomes a lifelong task that the individual must traverse in freedom and responsibility. . . . Only those who incorporate this ownmost and insuperable possibility in the form of a free and conscious running up [*Vorlaufen*] to death—and thus as an active feat of one's own freedom—raise themselves from . . . non-authenticity into the freedom of authentic self-being."[54] Rahner's Heiddegerian insight is that human beings often lose sight of their own freedom. One "may be like driftwood, and in a cowardly, lazy manner, he may regard himself as but the product of his age and environment. But his real duty is to accept his freedom willingly and without force, to love it and to have the courage to face it" (87).

Craigo-Snell elaborates Rahner's position in terms that will recall the concept of burdened agency: "Human beings find themselves in the middle of an already ongoing freedom that demands decisions and action. We have been burdened with an *imposed freedom* that we cannot discard. Yet we can choose how we regard and enact this freedom. . . . In facing our own death, we must decide how to understand and live out our own freedom, either as 'forced freedom or free liberty.'"[55] According to Robert Ochs, "Rahner's . . . approach to death as act comes from a conviction that everything in a person's existence should ultimately be act, should be freely affirmed. Man is basically defined by freedom. . . . Even man's freedom, which he discovers as a fact, must be freely assumed. It has to be taken up as a task. The imposed freedom must become free freedom."[56] In Heideggerian terms, will we finally grasp our authenticity?

Essentially, one's relationship to death reflects one's manner of living. "In death the soul achieves the consummation of its own personal self-affirmation, not merely passively suffering something which supervenes biologically, but through its own personal act" (30–31). Death "must be an active consummation from within . . . the achievement of total self-possession, a real effectuation of self, the fullness of freely produced personal reality" (31). At the same time, "inseparably and in a way which affects the whole human being, the death of man as the end of a material biological being is a destruction, a rupture, an accident which strikes man from without. . . . This simultaneity of fulfilment and emptiness, of actively achieved and passively suffered end, of full self-possession and of being completely dispossessed of self, may, for the moment be taken as a correct description of the phenomenon we call death" (40).

It must be noted that Rahner here has in view a highly abstract notion of death. He is not speaking about suicidal tendencies or taking one's dying into one's own hands. Rahner does not believe that death as an "act" occurs in a single moment (as, for example, in the deathbed tête-à-tête between man and God) but, rather, that it is "achieved through the act of the whole of life in such a manner that death is axiologically present all through human life. Man is enacting his death, as his own consummation, and in this way death is present in his actions, that is, in each of his free acts, in which he freely disposes of his whole person" (44).

Activity, Passivity, and Human Freedom

At times, Rahner's language seems to suggest that what is most important about the character of this act is that it is a self-conscious forging of one's basic identity. It is almost as if Rahner is proposing a radical self-assertion on the part of the individual, an existentialist act of self-creation that relies on individual will. Have we here arrived at Battin's "Stoic" view of death ("one's role should be as far as possible active, self-assertive, and responsible and may include ending one's own life"), only now in a Christian theological key?

While such a conclusion is tempting, it is ultimately misguided. For Rahner's understanding of the personal "act" of death is not ultimately about self-assertion but rather an act of self-surrender. To understand this, it is perhaps best to begin with an account of Christ's death. It is Rahner's contention that in his dying, Christ fundamentally changed death itself.

> The real miracle of Christ's death resides precisely in this: death which in itself can only be experienced as the advent of emptiness, as the im-

passe of sin, as the darkness of eternal night . . . and which "in itself" could be suffered, even by Christ himself, only as such a state of abandonment by God, now, through being embraced by the obedient "yes" of the Son, and while losing nothing of the horror of the divine abandonment that belongs to it, is transformed into something completely different, into the advent of God in the midst of that empty loneliness, and the manifestation of a complete, obedient surrender of the whole man to the holy God at the very moment when man seems lost and far removed from him. (71–72)

Through Christ's obedience, "the dreadful falling into the hands of the living God, which death must appear as a manifestation of sin, becomes in reality, 'Into Thy hands I commit my spirit'" (72).

Surrender is a peculiar mix of activity and passivity, an active release of self in trust of another.[57] As Craigo-Snell remarks of the crucifixion, "Jesus *acts* precisely in his powerlessness and passivity."[58] Notably, for Rahner, Jesus's death reveals not only the true nature of our own dying but also the very essence of human freedom: one can only become truly free by giving up the desire to grasp at freedom, and by surrendering in trust to the "nameless mystery which we call God."[59] Rahner notes that the redeemed Christian dies a "different death" from that of the sinner. Death no longer has the quality of being a penalty for sin, but rather, remaining a consequence of sin, it becomes an instrument of God "for our purification and testing" (67). The New Testament speaks of a "dying in the Lord" (Apoc 14:13; 1 Thess 4:13–18; 1 Cor 15:18) and a dying with Christ (2 Tim 2:11; Rom 6:8), which begins with baptism and faith, and continues as a lifelong process of *mortificatio* (Rom 6:6–14, 7:4–6, 8:2, 6–12), demonstrated publicly in the Church through sacraments of Eucharist and Unction (75).

What does this "dying with Christ" look like? According to Rahner, death "is faced rightly when it is entered upon by man as an act in which he surrenders himself fully and with unconditional openness to the disposal of the incomprehensible decision of God" (44). Such is the death of the martyrs, which "discloses *the essence* of Christian death" (101; emphasis added). The martyrs, in fact, evidence such utter freedom in surrender that they even have "love for death and courage for death" (87). Conversely, "mortal sin consists in the will to die autonomously, when death's open orientation toward God (which is contained in its obscurity) is not consented to" (44).

CONCLUSION: A SPIRITUALITY OF MARTYRDOM

This chapter began with Margaret Battin's claim that the "Christian" view of death, in contrast to the "Stoic" view, was characterized as hands-off and passive. A better way to think about the Christian view of agency in dying than this active-passive binary is in terms of a "spirituality of martyrdom," which also emphasizes the connection between patience, obedience, and active responsibility. This phrase, which was introduced by Servais Pinckaers, O.P., connects two important notions. First, it implies that moral theology is primarily concerned with the shape of the Christian life as a whole, what Pinckaers refers to as "spirituality,"[60] before it is concerned with concrete, particular decisions. "Spirituality," in this sense, situates the Christian standpoint in relation to the dominant cultural practices and social imaginaries, and points to how Christians can renarrate such things within the Christian story. As both Rahner and Pinckaers suggest, with respect to death and dying, the concept of martyrdom is precisely one locus for such generative activity to occur.

To be sure, martyrdom is a concept that will strike many contemporary readers as misguided, if not potentially dangerous. The theopolitical implications have been felt especially acutely since 9/11.[61] There are many noteworthy works dealing critically with important issues regarding the nature and purpose of martyrdom. These issues include debates about the prevalence of persecution in the early church, the psychological and spiritual motivations of early Christian martyrs, the conditions for official church designation as a martyr, and the relationship between the act of martyrdom and early Christian proclamation and self-identity. As important as each of these issues is, I am more interested at this point in how the work of Pinckaers, Rahner, and others[62] draws from the theological meaning of martyrdom to inform and influence moral and spiritual life in contemporary Western societies.

Pinckaers, for example, suggests "even if we are not threatened with death in the Western countries, we are all [still] called to give witness [*marturia*] to the Lord and to the Gospel in our daily actions and in our life in society" (4). Giving "witness" occurs through proclamation of the gospel and through obedient lives that testify to Christ's lordship. Therefore, martyrdom "does not represent one tiny spirituality among others; rather, it is written in the very heart of the Gospel."[63] Pinckaers notes the martyr's connection with Christ's humble self-giving (described by Paul as emptying, or *kenosis*, in Phil 2), in that the martyr is the one who is "obedient to the point of death" (8). "The first and principal element of Christian martyrdom . . . [is] the witness given to Christ, so complete that it extends to the acceptance of death" (38). Notably, however, the death here mentioned need not be strictly understood as being put to death. Pinckaers refers to Augustine, who "adds that a Christian can be a martyr in his bed, if he remains faithful to Christ in the face of disease and death, refusing the amulets and superstitions that some hold out to him." According to Augustine, "the principle element defining Christian martyrdom is not the suffering that one undergoes but the cause for which one accepts it. . . . Our suffering is not what makes us martyrs of God, but rather our justice" (Sermon 285). Pinckaers concludes, "The martyrs invite us, in our turn, to bear witness to our faith in Christ with intelligence and patience, faithfully and proudly, relying on the grace of the Spirit and on prayer more than on our own abilities and resources, whether personal or technical. [They invite us to bear witness] through every difficulty, contradiction, temptation, and humiliation that we may encounter, so that we too may prove to be good servants of divine Providence in the present world, good seeds planted in the soil of God for future harvests" (8).

Considering how the tradition of Roman Catholic moral theology envisions what it means for human beings to die and how they should imagine their own dying, I believe that the basic posture could be described as a "spirituality of martyrdom." The early Christian martyrs were recognized for the way in which they faced death openly, accepting death as an opportunity to surrender fully and unconditionally to God. They freely gave themselves over to it, thereby demonstrating a lived dependence on and trust in God's justice. Indeed, this posture can define any death that is faced by the believer. We will return to the notion of martyrdom, especially as it relates to the practices of the church and the formation of Christian identity in the final chapter of this book. It is through practices like baptism and Eucharist that one is prepared to make "obedience unto death," in the words of Rahner, the "axiological principle of one's life."

FOUR

Karl Barth on Agency in Dying

Accepting Creaturely Finitude

DEATH AND THE DOCTRINE OF CREATION

The theology of twentieth-century Swiss Protestant theologian Karl Barth provides a unique vantage point for considering agency in dying. Barth's theology considers the status of death and mortality within a universe understood as the good creation of a good God. Barth asks whether death is inherently evil—or whether it is only contingently so. Barth also explains the relationship between sin, guilt, and death. Ultimately, however, Barth is most interesting because of how he describes the shape of the Christian ethical stance, posture, or response to death and mortality. In other words, how should human beings relate to the brute fact of mortality, on the one hand, and to their own mortality, on the other?

Barth offers a self-consciously modern approach to theology in general and to theological anthropology in particular.[1] He was not overly concerned with offering an apologetic response to the challenges confronting traditional Christianity in the guise of evolutionary science, Enlightenment rationalism, historical relativism, or biblical criticism. Barth was certainly aware of these intellectual movements, taking them seriously as he formulated his own dogmatic theology, but his interest lay elsewhere than building walls to protect orthodoxy from modernity or building "eternal covenants" to ensure their mutual coexistence.[2] Rather, Barth "in the end, was seeking to understand what it means to be orthodox *under the conditions of modernity*."[3]

This is especially important in light of the stark challenges modern thought has presented for traditional doctrines of creation. As Katherine Sonderegger has pointed out, in the nineteenth and twentieth centuries, theologians treating the doctrine of creation "could hardly speak with the confident tones of earlier eras. From the rise of modern astronomy to the carbon-dating of our earth and the development of present-day animal species, the genesis of all things from God has found itself in the midst of pitched battles over the place and cogency of Christian doctrine in an intellectual climate dominated by the exact sciences and driven by fear of them."[4] In light of these challenges, modern theology has taken up with exceptional vigor the question of the "natural"—in other words, "when God created all that is, just what is it that he made?"[5]

It is axiomatic in Christian theology that creation, though marred by sin and evil, is fundamentally good. Sonderegger suggests that a "fundamental analysis of the creaturely"[6] affords us insights into which aspects of creaturely existence are rightly to be lamented and which are more properly to be celebrated. This is significant for a theological understanding of death and dying. Traditional understandings of creation consistently denied that God had created a world marked by death and dying, whether in the human or animal world. In a post-Darwinian world, however, it becomes impossible even for proponents of theistic evolution to deny the reality of death before the fall of humankind into sin.[7] Death via predation, it seems, not only occurred but was a central mechanism of human development and growth. As a distinctively "modern" theologian, Barth's answer to the question of death is especially relevant.

The second reason for turning to Barth's theology is that it expresses, borrowing a phrase from philosopher Stanley Cavell, "an acknowledgement of human limitation which does not leave us chafed by our own skin."[8] It does so through a full-throated theological articulation of the nature and significance of human finitude. Barth was not the first to consider the finitude of creaturely existence as a divine gift,[9] but he was able to affirm the goodness of creaturely finitude in a particularly clear and forceful way. It stands to reason that if we are able to appreciate how exactly Barth understood death and mortality in relation to creaturely finitude, we might place ourselves in a position to articulate an ethical stance from which to consider our own approaches to dying. This vision of the goodness of finitude provides powerful critical leverage over against what was earlier described as the "Baconian project" in modern medicine.

The broad contours of Barth's view of human mortality are present in the following quotation, found near the end of his treatment of theological anthropology:

> If hope in Christ is a real liberation for natural death, this rests on the fact that by divine appointment death as such belongs to the life of the creature and is thus necessary to it. Adamic man was created a *psuchen zosan* (1 Cor 15:45), and therefore a being which has only its own span of time. His definitive relationship to God as the end and goal of human life demands that this life itself should be defined and therefore limited. On this limit there is made in its favour the divine decision which is the substance of the New Testament message of salvation. On this limit it was made in the life of the man Jesus. He had to die, to submit to the judgment of God and thus restore the right of God and that of man. "Except a corn of wheat fall into the ground and die, it abideth alone; but if it die, it bringeth forth much fruit" (John 12:24). We cannot try to love and maintain finally and absolutely our life in this time; otherwise we shall lose it. We must give it up in order to save it (Matt 16:25).... If we did not have to do with the definitive end of human life, we should not have to do with its resurrection and definitive co-existence with that of God.... We are invited to accept the limit of the life which He has rescued, and therefore to acquiesce in the fact that we must have an end, and to set our hope wholly and utterly in Him. (*Church Dogmatics* [*CD*] III.2, 639)

Barth's position is not straightforward. He is willing to call death "natural" and to affirm its belonging to the creaturely existence of the human being. Mortality is a "necessary" precondition of both the covenantal relationship between God and humanity and the saving work of Jesus Christ. At the same time, however, he suggests that a "real liberation" must take place for the naturalness of death to become a possibility.

In what follows, I will unpack each of these aspects of Barth's understanding of death and dying. Although Barth opens up possibilities for affirming the finitude of human life, he does not evade the harshness and apparent evilness of death. In the next section, I will consider whether and to what degree Barth considers death to be an evil. The answer to this question is complicated by the fact that both "death" and "evil," in Barth's usage, are terms that must be considered dialectically. Barth makes a distinction between death "as it meets us" (what I call empirical death) and death as the natural limit to life (what I call natural death). Barth also makes a distinction between "nothingness" (i.e., *das Nichtige*, Barth's preferred term for evil), which only exists as that which is definitely rejected by God, and the "shadow side" of creation, that which is sad and difficult but nevertheless belongs to the goodness of the world. After explaining why empirical death belongs to *das Nichtige* and is therefore wholly evil, I will explain how Christ's death frees human beings for natural death and how, correlatively, death becomes an instrument of divine grace. I will then return to the concept of natural death, explaining in greater detail its biblical roots, as well as its implications for theological anthropology. I will show how Barth sees natural death as a precondition of certain creaturely goods, including temporality, historical particularity, and subjectivity. I will then conclude by considering the ethical implications of Barth's understanding of death and mortality.

TAKING DEATH SERIOUSLY
(BUT NOT TOO SERIOUSLY)

Death as Evil: Sin, Guilt, and Judgment

If Barth finds a way to accept and even affirm the limited and mortal nature of human existence it is not because he fails to take death seriously. In fact, Barth adamantly argues that death must be seen for what it is: "the abyss of our negation" (*CD* III.2, 588). There is no downplaying death's totality and utter finality (compare 2 Sam 14:14; Job 7:9, 16:22). "When we die, all things and we ourselves come to an end" (*CD* III.2, 588). Barth repeatedly denies that death is merely the transition of the soul from a bodily to a bodyless state. That is merely a pagan wish. "Whatever existence in death may mean, it cannot consist in a continuation of life in time. One day we shall have had our life. . . . We shall one day *have been*" (*CD* III.2, 589; emphasis added). In Old Testament terms, if we may speak of one's "existence" in Sheol, it can only be an existence of a faint and shadowy sort. Death is an "alien," "menacing," and "potent force" (*CD* III.2, 590), which confronts us all "as an incomprehensible, inexplicable and unassailable reality" (*CD* III.2, 588). This is why the Old Testament uses the images of the pit, the ocean, and the wilderness to evoke death. These are the three "nonworlds" that confront humankind as the border and limit of the space of the living. They also metaphorically represent the "chaos" that opposes God's ordering of creation (*CD* III.2, 591). Death, understood as a menacing chaotic force, even infringes on life in the form of sickness, cursedness, and loneliness.

That death opposes life is reason enough to consider it an evil, but to understand the real evil of death, according to Barth, we must consider it under a covenantal perspective. In the Old Testament, the evil in death is that it threatens the divine covenant between God and humanity with "relationlessness." Those in Sheol are cut off from the land of the living, from the worshipping community, and from God (see Ps 6:3, 30:9, 115:17, 88:11–12; Isa 38:18–19).

Theologically speaking, relationlessness "is true already here and now" (*CD* III.2, 592) because of sin, for sin is essentially the human rejection of God's covenantal love and grace. There is, then, a connection between sin, guilt, and death. As sinners, we are guilty of this rejection and deserve the "judgment" of being handed over to it. It is this guilt that makes death so terrifying, for the moment of death seals our guilt as it is and therefore concludes our life as finally a sinful one. Death is the "seal and fulfillment of man's negation" (*CD* III.2, 625) because the God who confronts us at our death "can only justly affirm" the negation that we have already chosen for ourselves. Barth is adamant that *this* death, the death of the sinner under the judgment of God, is most decidedly not natural. "Death as it actually meets us" (*CD* III.2, 597) is "not a part of man's nature as God created it" (*CD* III.2, 600) but rather "the great mark of the unnatural state in which we exist" (*CD* III.2, 601).

From this conclusion, two observations follow. First, what is unnatural is not the fact that life is temporally limited, that it will one day come to an end. Rather, the unnatural thing is the sinful state of existence that is sealed at the moment of death and that merits divine judgment. Second, when Barth speaks about the death of the sinner, he quite often qualifies it with a phrase like "as it actually meets us" (*CD* III.2, 597) or "as it actually encounters us men" (*CD* III.2, 596). This phrase is one of the keys to interpreting Barth's understanding of human dying. We might call the death of the sinner de facto death, or, following G. C. Berkouwer, "empirical death."[10]

"Empirical," it must be noted, does not mean "inferred from general experience." It is not a matter of inductive reasoning. As a thoroughly Christological thinker, Barth's understanding of creation, and especially his theological anthropology, takes Jesus Christ to be "the one point at the centre of creation where the Creator-creature relationship is revealed."[11] Barth repeatedly warns against presuming "abstract" knowledge about the world or about humanity which may be gained apart from the event of revelation in Jesus Christ. In line with Barth's theological epistemology, therefore, we would do well to remember that even Barth's notion of "empirical death" is Christological. Perhaps unsurprisingly, then, it is to the death of Jesus Christ that we should look for insight into the nature of death. That death is *empirically* the sign of judgment is revealed ultimately in the fact that Jesus died on our behalf and suffered death as the actual judgment of God.

Death and Nothingness

Barth never develops a "doctrine of evil" because the task of dogmatics is the proclamation and explication of the gospel. Theology does not dwell on evil in the abstract but rather witnesses to the "Creator, creature and their co-existence, and the intrusion upon them of the undeniable reality of" evil (*CD* III.3, 365). Because the proper focus of theology is precisely on Christ's victory over evil, the Christian rightly views evil as that which is opposed by God, as that which God rejects.

Barth makes a distinction between creation's "shadow side" and "evil" (Barth's preferred term is *das Nichtige*, nothingness). The former is distinct from evil insofar as it is positively willed by God; the latter is wholly opposed to the will of God and only exists as that which is rejected by God.[12] Physical and biological mortality, as miserable and terrible as it can be, belongs to the shadow side of creation. It is not wholly evil. What is evil, according to Barth, is the spiritual death that results from the wholly deserved judgment of God on sinful humanity, which is to say, "death in God abandonment." To make this point clearer, let us explore these notions a bit more deeply.

In the section titled "The Yes of God the Creator" (§42), Barth stresses the unqualified goodness of creation, including "the limits of . . . creatureliness." Barth leaves no ambiguity: "God the Creator did not say No, nor Yes and No, but Yes to what He created" (*CD* III.1, 330). It is here that Barth distinguishes between "two contradictory aspects" (*CD* III.1, 375) within creation. On the one side, there is all that is beautiful and pleasant and sweet, all that rightly calls forth a joyous and grateful response. It is easy to affirm creation's "brighter side" (*CD* III.1, 370) as worthy of divine affirmation, but this does not exhaust creation's goodness. For there is also an element of creation that rightly calls for weeping and lament (*CD* III.1, 373) — the "shadow side" — which is nevertheless willed and desired by God. Barth does not specify which experiences and phenomena belong to this shadow side but does not hesitate to use terms such as "need," "peril," and "misery" to describe it. Nevertheless, Barth insists, the shadow side of creation stands with its brighter side under the unequivocal "yes" of God the Creator.

Barth's understanding of *das Nichtige* is basically Augustinian (evil as a deficiency that is parasitic on the good), but his actualistic ontology shifts his account in a more historicist and Christological framework.[13] Instead of a "great chain of Being," Barth's dominating metaphor is that of "covenant." It is the covenant of God with humankind enacted in Jesus Christ that forms the basis for Barth's holding together of the "brighter side" and the "shadow side" of creation under the divine yes. "For in [Jesus Christ] God has made Himself the Subject of both aspects of creaturely existence. And having made it His own in Jesus Christ, He has affirmed it in its totality, reconciling its inner antithesis in His own person" (*CD* III.3, 296). Barth's supralapsarian Christology means that creation as a whole is always already enveloped within the saving will of God — in both beauty and tragedy, harmony and dissonance, brightness and shadow.[14]

Creation, then, in its totality, is good because it is ordered toward the goal of the covenant between God and humankind. Because God's covenant transcends these "two contradictory aspects" (*CD* III.1, 375), it confirms both without being "exhausted" by either, unifying them in a totality by taking the creaturely contradiction to Himself. Barth makes the connection with mortality explicit: "Primarily and supremely [God] has made [the contradiction of creation] His own, and only then caused it to be reflected in the life of the creature.... Before life greeted us and death menaced us, He was the Lord of life and death, and bound them both in a bundle" (*CD* III.1, 380). Because "the joy and the misery of life have their foundation in the will of God" (*CD* III.1, 376), one should not wish "to elude the shadow" entirely, for to do so would be to deny what God has affirmed.

Barth's aesthetic account of creation is reflected in his description of his appreciation for his favorite composer, Wolfgang Amadeus Mozart.[15] "[Mozart] knew something about creation in its total goodness.... He heard the harmony of creation to which the shadow also belongs but in which the shadow is not darkness, deficiency is not defeat, sadness cannot become despair, trouble cannot degenerate into tragedy and infinite melancholy is not ultimately forced to claim undisputed sway. Thus the cheerfulness in this harmony is not without its limits. But *the light shines all the more brightly because it breaks forth from the shadow*. The sweetness is also bitter and cannot therefore cloy. *Life does not fear death but knows it well*" (*CD* III.3, 298; emphases added). In short, Mozart's music is beautiful because it is *true*, and this is the case for two reasons: First, Mozart neither ignores nor evades the difficult and unhappy aspects of creaturely existence. Mozart's genius lies in his ability to "translate into music . . . real life in all its discord."[16] Second, however, Mozart understood that refusing to ignore dissonance does not mean holding it in equilibrium with consonance and resolution. "What occurs in Mozart is rather a glorious upsetting of the balance, a turning in which the light rises and the shadows fall, though without disappearing, in which joy overtakes sorrow without extinguishing it, in which the Yea rings louder than the ever-present Nay."[17] For all of these reasons, Barth affirms Mozart's music as a "parable of the kingdom."[18]

The shadow, however, must be sharply distinguished from evil, which Barth calls *das Nichtige*.[19] In distinction from the former, the latter cannot be understood as beautiful or good in any way. *Das Nichtige* does not refer to the necessary limitations that accompany creaturely existence and that are therefore to be accepted as the shadow that makes the light all the more appealing. *Das Nichtige* names that which God conclusively opposes and rejects in the creation and redemption of all that is. *Das Nichtige* is an "alien factor" (*CD* III.3, 289), "a real enemy" (301) and an "adversary with whom no compromise is possible" (302).

What, then, ought we to make of death? Is it an expression of the power of *das Nichtige*, of the evil chaos that can only be rejected and overcome by God in Christ, or does it belong to the shadow side of creation, a sad and lamentable but nevertheless good and appropriate feature of creaturely existence? The answer is, it depends on what one means by "death." There are indeed moments when Barth seems to indicate that death is best understood as an expression of *das Nichtige*. As "the intolerable, life-destroying thing to which all suffering hastens as its goal, as the ultimate irruption and triumph of that alien power which annihilates creaturely existence and thus discredits and disclaims the Creator" (*CD* III.3, 312), death is utterly evil. What Barth calls "real death" in his treatment of evil is "empirical death," the death of the sinner. When Barth speaks of "*real* death"—as when he speaks of "real sin" and "real evil"—he refers explicitly to that which is "in opposition to the totality of God's creation" (*CD* III.3, 310). As we will see, however, Barth distinguishes this "real death" from the "mere matter of dying as the natural termination of life" (*CD* III.3, 312).

DEATH AS A FORM GRACE TAKES

Death as the Sign of Judgment

But here, another question arises. How is it that Barth can speak of a form of death that is in no way "empirical" for us? If death is the sign of divine judgment and if this judgment even fell on the Savior, what business have we speaking about a natural death? Barth admits that this other form of death remains "unfathomably and inaccessibly concealed beneath the unnatural and even anti-natural guise in which it now comes to us" (*CD* III.2, 598). Nevertheless, Barth claims that death may also be understood as the natural limit of human life. This conclusion is not made on the basis of general experience but rather on the basis of the covenant that is revealed and realized precisely through the death of Jesus Christ (*CD* III.2, 614).

In the death of Jesus Christ, God executed a negative judgment on human sin. As sinners we rightly fear death because we fear judgment: it is a terrible thing to fall into the hands of the living God (Heb 10:31)! Critically, however, this God who confronts us in death is not an "abstract concept of deity" but rather the very God who "has graciously undertaken to suffer the judgment of death in the death of [Jesus Christ] and thus to release us from it" (*CD* III.2, 626). It is significant that, for Barth, empirical death is the "sign of divine judgment" and not the "divine judgment" itself. The divine judgment that is merited by the sinful existence of the human is death in God abandonment—and there is one person of whom we may say that he died this death. "*Eloi, Eloi, lama sabachtani?*" (Matt 27:46). Because Jesus has actually suffered the judgment of God, "dying no longer has to be this dying, the suffering of punishment which [sinful humans] have deserved, *but only its sign*" (*CD* III.2, 600; emphasis added). Because Jesus has died this death, "those who believe in Jesus can no longer look at their death as though it were in front of them. It is behind them" (*CD* III.2, 621). Death, then, may be the inescapable limit to the human being, but it is a limit that itself is limited by God. God is therefore in very truth the boundary of the death that bounds us. What awaits us at our limit, then, is not our annihilation but the gracious God. To approach death, then, allows for "greater contact with grace."[20]

At Our End—God:
The Role of Death in Barth's Romans Commentary

Perhaps the best way to elaborate the logic that makes death the point of contact with divine grace is to turn to Barth's earlier writings. Death plays a central but seldom recognized role in the theology of Barth's early period and, especially, in the second edition of his commentary on the *Epistle to the Romans*.[21] In *Romans* II, death is at once a decisive no to human presumption, the very means of deliverance from sinful existence, and the place of encounter with divine grace.

Upon encountering *Romans* II for the first time, the reader will likely be struck by a sense of disorientation or uneasiness, as if walking through a funhouse on a tightrope. Such a reader might be encouraged to find out that this is precisely the intended effect of Barth's forceful rhetoric. Barth desired to leave the reader "suspended in the air" with "no standing-place" but the absolute miracle of divine grace (*Romans* II, 94, 163). Explaining why Barth sought to inculcate this attitude in the reader—and how he did it—will, perhaps surprisingly, bring us at least part of the way to an understanding of the meaning and importance of death in Barth's early theology.

Barth's commentary, described by one of his contemporaries as a "bombshell on the playground of the theologians," was intended as a disruption.[22] It was written during an early period of Barth's career when he was becoming increasingly dissatisfied with the dominant liberal theology of his day, and it was especially motivated by his shocked horror at the ease with which most of his former teachers had provided religious justification for their support of the war policy of German emperor Wilhelm II.[23] At the heart of Barth's break with liberal theology was the issue of theological epistemology. Specifically, what is the role of human experience in the knowledge of God and of humanity in light of God? Many German Christians, like Martin Rade and Wilhelm Herrmann, had appealed to the almost-supernatural experience of unity with which the German people met the prospect of war as evidence for its divine authorization. But such an interpretation was so far afield from Barth's own "'experience' of God in Jesus"[24] that it called into question the usefulness of the very category of experience as "an adequate ground and starting-point for theology."[25] What was most blatantly missing from these liberal theologians, according to Barth, was any discernable element of self-criticism regarding the knowledge of God. It was with *Romans* II, and its radical element of self-critique, that Barth's break with liberal theology was brought to its clearest and most powerful expression.

It is within this context that we should seek to understand one of Barth's recurring metaphors in *Romans* II: the "line of death" (*Todeslinie*). In the first instance, the "line of death" fulfills the largely negative and critical role of marking the impassable boundary (*Grenz*) between human beings and God. "The Being and Action of God are and remain wholly different from the being and action of men. The line which separates here from there cannot be crossed: it is the line of death (*Todeslinie*)" (*Romans* II, 111).

In a broken world, "everything that occurs . . . is bent under the judgement of God and awaits His affirmation" (*Romans* II, 111). The decisive "judgment" (*Krisis*) of God declares an "infinite qualitative distinction" between time and eternity, between the created world and the uncreated God (*Romans* II, 10). With regard to epistemology, this means that God and humanity do not stand, whether near or far from each other, along a single continuum that might give the human some point of contact (*Kontaktpunkt*) for recognizing the divine. Barth was convinced, in the words of Bruce McCormack, that "the way taken by a person who seeks to know God will, to a large extent, determine what kind of God one arrives at, or even whether what is arrived at is God at all."[26] In a key passage Barth proclaims,

> We suppose that we know what we are saying when we say "God." We assign to Him the highest place in our world: and in doing so we place Him fundamentally on one line with ourselves and with things. . . . We dare to deck ourselves out as His companions, patrons, advisers, and commissioners. We confound time with eternity. . . . *Secretly we are ourselves the masters in this relationship.* We are not concerned with God, but with our own requirements, to which God must adjust Himself. . . . And so, when we set God upon the throne of the world, we mean by God ourselves. . . . God Himself is not acknowledged as God and what is called "God" is in fact man. (*Romans* II, 40; emphasis original)

The importance of the sentence in italics in this quotation should not be overlooked. If God is to be known *as God*, then God cannot at any point become merely the *object* of human knowledge; God must also remain the *Subject* in the encounter between God and humanity.[27]

How is this possible? In *Romans* II, Barth gives a twofold answer. The first has to do with the event of revelation in the life history of Jesus Christ, and the second has to do with the event of revelation in the life of the believer. Both invoke death, but here, we will focus on the latter.

In explicating the event of revelation, Barth draws attention to the need for repentance and conversion. A sinful individual cannot straightforwardly receive revelation. No, revelation "requires a new subject" (*Romans* II, 62) which it also creates: the "Old Man" must be put to death so the "New Man" can come into existence. God remains subject in the event of revelation because revelation occurs only insofar as the recipient undergoes an *Aufhebung* in which her identity is dissolved in Christ's death only to reestablish in his resurrection. But without death, there is no resurrection: "By dissolving us, He establishes us; by killing us, He gives us life" (*Romans* II, 61).

It is precisely because our fundamental sin is "our drunken blurring of the distance which separates us from God" that human beings need to be taken to their absolute limit to be judged as those who nevertheless fall short of God. It is precisely in this "going to the limit," the negation of every human possibility, that reveals the infinite qualitative distinction and opens up the space for God to be recognized as God (*Romans* II, 76, 202).[28] Thus for Barth, somewhat paradoxically, "grace presupposes the line of death by which all concrete human conspicuousness is bounded absolutely. This line is, however, in God's sight the line of life, since it assumes the final negation which alone contains the affirmation of God" (*Romans* II, 138).

"Beyond the barrier at which we stand is—God" (*Romans* II, 93). To approach the "line of death," then, is not simply to approach the utter limit (*Grenz*) of human possibility but is also to approach the place of the uniquely divine possibility of grace. This is precisely what we witness in Jesus's death. Jesus did not die as a "hero or leader of men." Whereas the primal couple sought to be "like God" (*sicut Deus*), Jesus sacrifices "every claim to genius and every human heroic or aesthetic or psychic possibility" before God. In this negation, a space is opened up as it were for the gracious action of God. Therefore, "in [Jesus] we behold the faithfulness of God in the depths of Hell. The Messiah is the end of mankind, and here also God is found faithful" (*Romans* II, 97).

Barth's understanding of death in *Romans* II has implications. The limit against which humanity rebelled "in Adam," which subsequently became for all humanity a curse, is thus given back to humanity as the concrete form grace takes. "Our life is confronted with a steep precipice, towering above us, hemming us in on every side, and on it are hewn the words: *All things come to an end*. And yet in all negativity there is no point which does not bear witness to the summit. . . . Death never occurs but it calls attention to our participation in the Life of God and to that relationship of His with us which is not broken by sin" (*Romans* II, 170). The believer, then, is freed to affirm the limited and contingent nature of creaturely existence. When this happens, a dramatic reversal occurs: "Death is deprived of its power. When we recognize that in suffering and brokenness it is *God* whom we encounter, that we have been cast up against Him and bound to Him, that we have been dissolved by Him and uplifted by Him, then tribulation worketh *probation* of faith, and faith discovers God to be the Originator of all things, and awaits all from Him" (*Romans* II, 157; emphasis original).

The event of revelation does this. It dissolves the sinner to reestablish her in light of God's faithfulness. This divine *Aufhebung* of the human being demonstrates a striking fact. Death, understood as the inescapable confrontation with the limited nature of human existence, is a presupposition of divine grace. The human being must be taken to her utter limit and must undergo the negation of all merely human possibilities to be shown that it is precisely at her limit that God remains God.

Death as the Gracious End of the Sinner

Having considered Barth's dialectical approach to death in *Romans* II, let us turn to a related construal from his later writings. In *Church Dogmatics* III.I, Barth returns to the theme of death as the precondition of grace in his exegesis of the second creation story and the fall of Adam. In this section, he reflects on the "tree of life," noting that the biblical text is relatively silent regarding its nature and significance. Whereas Genesis 3:22 suggests a relationship between the tree and unending life, God offers no "explicit promise in connexion [*sic*] with it" (*CD* III.1, 256). Although the tree of life is in the midst of the Garden of Eden and although there was no prohibition against eating from it, Adam never seems to have done so. Given that God was directly and intimately upholding Adam's life, his doing so would perhaps have been superfluous. The "tree of life" seems to gain importance only after Adam partakes of the "tree of the knowledge of good and evil." Why is this? As Barth explains, the particular wickedness of this act was in the grasping after the ability to determine right and wrong, which wholly belongs to God as the rightful Judge and Creator. Adam should have desired to receive "good and evil" from God's own hand (*CD* III.1, 260) and not to exalt himself to a position of fellow judgeship, as if to either confirm or disconfirm the judgment of God (*CD* III.1, 261). In his attempt to define right and wrong, Adam was essentially acting as if he were creator rather than creature. "But this is a responsibility which exceeds his capacity. He will necessarily collapse under the burden no less than if he were given the whole globe to carry" (*CD* III.1, 261). It is worth noting that the death that follows is less an externally imposed punishment than an intrinsic and necessary result of failing to cleave to the source of life. "Choosing and deciding for himself, he must now be the fountain of life himself. But he is unable to be the fountain of life himself. Hence he can only forfeit his life and die." Placed in this position, the creature "cannot continue as a creature. It is poison for any being to have to stand in the place of God" (*CD* III.1, 262).

Once the nature of this first grasping became clear, it would have been a terrible calamity for Adam to have similarly grasped after life—which, in any case, like "good and evil," was to be received from God's own hand. Here, we return to the significance of Genesis 3:22: had Adam grasped after this tree, he would, "in some sense, [be] deifying his self-merited fate, giving to death itself . . . [the] character of eternal life, and thus delivering himself up to eternal death" (*CD* III.1, 257). Given this danger, limitation of life is not only a natural result of turning away from the source of life but also a gracious restriction of the power of the human being to oppose and reject the limits placed on it by God. "[Adam's] only hope, the only guarantee in face of death, is that grasping at the tree of life should be made impossible to him; that the matter should simply end in death, that he should be allowed to die in order that, dying, he may at least fulfill without resistance the will of God as he must encounter it after his transgression, in order that in death at least he should be in [God's] hand, and therefore should not be rejected, but should have his hope in God" (*CD* III.1, 284).[29] A boundary must be set to the life of the sinner. Immortality would be a disaster for sinful human beings. Death is a severe mercy.

DEATH AS A NATURAL END

Empirical versus Natural Death

We have seen that for Barth, death must be taken quite seriously as the sign of judgment. Empirical death declares an unequivocal no against sinful humanity, threatening separation from God and eternal damnation. We have also seen, however, that the very God whom we fear in death is the God who has chosen not to be without us by becoming one with us in Jesus Christ and by suffering the consequences of the divine no on our behalf. Death is therefore both the terrible consequence of sin and the locus of salvation. It is only through death that we can be saved from death, for without death, there is no resurrection.

Barth goes further. Not only are we saved *from* empirical death, but we are saved "*for* natural death" (*CD* III.2, 638; emphasis added). Jesus has died the empirical death for us (*pro nobis*), "death now wears a guise in which we can look it in the face. We can now face it as a natural prospect" (*CD* III.2, 638). Although the two actually coincide in the majority of the biblical references to death and dying, Barth does not believe that our empirical death and our natural end necessarily and intrinsically belong together. But how does Barth distinguish between empirical and natural death? In the course of drawing them apart, Barth makes two sorts of arguments: an argument based on scripture and an argument based on the incarnation.

First, although he recognizes that he must rely on "a narrower compass of biblical demonstration" (*CD* III.2, 633), Barth believes that the scriptures themselves provide evidence of a more benign form of death. Part of the complication is that the Old and New Testaments almost always refer to death in the harsher sense. There is, however, another form of death in the Bible, what David called "the way of all earth" (1 Kings 2:3) and Balaam called "the death of the upright" (Num 23:10). Barth argues that one can see glances in the Old Testament of deaths not primarily characterized by judgment and curse. When Moses died, he was buried by YHWH Himself. Enoch seems to have been translated directly from existence into nonexistence as if "unawares." Elijah was taken to God on a chariot of fire. These examples are obviously exceptions to the rule, but they reveal—not as a human possibility but by the grace of God—the possibility of a natural end.

These scriptural and exegetical arguments, however, cannot stand on their own. At best, Barth understands them to be elaborations of the truth revealed in the death of Jesus Christ. Although empirical death and natural death do indeed coincide in the death of Jesus, Barth argues that they need not have. "Since He was neither sinful nor guilty . . . His human life might have ended in quite a different way. . . . In His human person there is manifested a human existence whose finitude is not intrinsically identical with bondage to that other death" (*CD* III.2, 629). Empirical death is thereby "set at a certain distance" from death understood as the divinely appointed end. Jesus was fully human and therefore he was mortal, able to die. But he "did not have to stand under the judgment of God or suffer the death of a reprobate" (*CD* III.2, 630). This proves that "the finitude of temporal existence obviously does not necessarily imply that we stand under the wrath of

God" (*CD* III.2, 630). Furthermore, if Christ had not been mortal, he would not have been able to die on our behalf. "And if His dying—in virtue of what it was as His—is the sum total of the good which God has shown to the world, how can we dare to understand man's mortality as something intrinsically negative and evil" (*CD* III.2, 630)?

The Goodness of Creaturely Finitude

The final judgment Barth makes is this: the "finitude of our being belongs to our God-given nature" (*CD* III.2, 627). As the previous pages should make clear, this judgment was hard won. It was not blithely put forth on the basis of general experience. It was not a simple denial of the evilness of death. The goodness of our finitude can only be known in light of the saving death of Jesus Christ. Once the possibility of a natural death has been established, however—once the temporal finitude of human life has been counted among the things that God created when God created the world—we may then inquire into the particular goods associated with living a finite life. In what sense can we count our mortality and even our death as a gift? Can it be accepted? Can it be embraced?

The first thing to establish is that natural death, as opposed to empirical death, is defined in terms of *creaturely* finitude rather than relationlessness. What, then, does it mean to be a creature? Barth's programmatic statement in this regard is "creation is the external basis of the covenant" and "the covenant is the internal basis of creation." To be a creature, then, is to be set in relation to the covenant between God and humanity, which finds its fulfillment in Jesus Christ. As the first act of God that "contains in itself the beginning of time" (*CD* III.1, 42), creation temporally precedes the fulfillment of the covenant. The whole point (telos) of creation, however, is to "set the stage for the story of the covenant of grace" (*CD* III.1, 44). Creation is not a neutral occurrence: it is itself ordered toward the redemption of humankind in Jesus Christ.

Because creation is ordered toward covenant, we are also able to say that creaturely limits are ordered toward that same goal. For example, discussing Genesis 1, Barth likens the firmament to a "theatre of life" eminently suitable for human dwelling. There would be no theater, however, without the "establishment of a boundary . . . the willing and creating of

[a] barrier" in the division of the waters above from the waters below (*CD* III.1, 133), as well as God's limiting of the sea on the third day of creation (*CD* III.1, 149). These boundaries set the stage for the covenantal telos of creation. In Barth's theological anthropology, boundaries (*die Grenzen*) are not primarily negative restrictions of humanity and human freedom but rather a necessary delimiting of the creature in all her particularity and individuality.

For Barth, to be a creature of God cannot be a curse. Regarding the sixth day of creation (Gen 1:24–31), Barth notes that humankind is created on the same day as the other land-dwelling creatures and are therefore, in some way, of a piece with them in their creaturehood (*CD* III.1, 178). As a result, human beings should not be overly eager to view themselves as superior to other animals. In fact, it seems human beings have something to learn from the wider sphere of creation about what it means to live *as a creature*:

> If it is true that man is more noble than these creatures, it is also true that he has just as much need of them as of all that went before, whereas they for their part have no need of him whatever. . . . The creature [in fact] precedes man in a self-evident praise of its Creator, in the natural fulfillment of the destiny given to it at its creation, in the actual humble recognition and confirmation of its creatureliness. It also precedes him in the fact that it does not forget but maintains its animal nature, with its dignity and also its limitation, and thus asks man whether and to what extent the same can be said of him. (*CD* III.1, 177)

Genesis 2 confirms the creaturely solidarity proclaimed in Genesis 1. If, in the first creation story, humans and animals are created *on the same day*, in the second, both are "*formed of dust*, animated by God and destined to return to dust and non-existence" (*CD* III.1, 238; emphasis added). The Hebrew term for "dust" (`aphar*) has a range of meanings. Literally, it refers to dry debris or loose earth. Under this aspect, it indicates a "strong emphasis on [human] creatureliness. . . . As far as his body is concerned, man [`*adam*] is of the earth [`*adamah*]" (*CD* III.1, 243). That human beings stand in an organic and natural connection with the earth is, on one level, a somewhat unremarkable view for an agrarian people group to hold. The ancient Hebrews would have understood the earth as the source of their subsistence and would know that what returns to the earth further contributes to its fecundity. To be "of the earth" in this sense, then, need not be lamented. Figuratively, however, ʿ*aphar* can also denote what is lowly, fragile, and even worthless. Dust, it might be pointed out, insofar as it is dry and loose, is not associated with arable climates. As it is not particularly productive of life, it is also associated with death. In the Old Testament, the term ʿ*aphar* is used metaphorically, to refer to a corpse (Ps 30:9) or to the grave itself (Ps 22:29; Gen 3:19). Taken at face value, one might assume that this means that it is something to be despised. Although such an interpretation would be a mistake, it carries the following grain of truth: the goodness of the material world is not an intrinsic feature but rather a result of God's always already relating to it. According to Barth, "the whole goodness of human creatureliness consists in what God made of this material and what He has in mind for it. It does not, therefore, lie in the material [itself]" (*CD* III.1, 245). This is even true of the human being, whose life, Genesis 2:7 tells us, depends on the direct impartation from God of the "breath of life." The "dust" is worthless apart from God, but it is never *apart from God*. This all points to the following conclusion: human existence, in all its bodily earthiness, is not a condition to be overcome but a gift to be received with thanksgiving. What is lowly in itself is exalted as it is encountered by God. "Because *as the creature of God* he is distinct from God, it cannot in any sense be a humiliation for him to be what he is" (*CD* III.1, 243; emphasis added).

In light of the death of Jesus Christ, we can go even further. We may affirm death (in the sense of the temporal limitation of life) both as a gracious "delimiting" of the individual's life in time, which gives it its particular shape and definition and as a sign of divine providence. In *CD* III.4 (§56), Barth offers a more positive interpretation that takes mortality to be the most conspicuous but by no means the only form of limitation graciously given to the human creature by God. These limitations are the concrete forms by which God delimits each of us as individual beings: "Limitation as decreed by God means circumscription, definition, and therefore determination. Only the void is undefined and therefore unlimited. Differentiating the creature from Himself, God limits it to be His creature and thus gives it its specific and genuine reality" (*CD* III.4, 567). God also limits us in this gracious way by placing each person in his or her own historical era, geographical location, and so forth. Every particularity is a limitation, but it is the particularity of our lives that lends them their very reality.

Further, according to Barth, the limitation of human life stands as "a sign and testimony of the divine world-governance" (*CD* III.3, 227). Barth gives four reasons: First, by presenting a challenge to our notions of self-sufficiency and self-mastery our finitude testifies to the Lordship of God. For in our natality and mortality "it is made clear that to live is something which I myself cannot take, or give, or maintain. . . . I am indebted to a power which ordained that I should live within the limits laid down not by myself but by that power" (*CD* III.3, 230). Second, in the "once-and-for-allness" lent to our life by the brackets of life and death, our finitude testifies to the uniqueness of God. Third, our life bracketed by birth and death comprises a single history in which one's freedom, as real as it is, is enclosed by the "severity and . . . mercy" (*CD* III.3, 233) of God and therefore testifies that God is the rightful judge of one's life. Finally, in ascending from birth and descending toward death, there takes place in our lives in nuce the very dynamic of all world history. All of this means that each and every one of us bears within our mortal lives a sign and testimony of God's faithfulness and preservation, whether we realize it or not.

CONCLUSION: KARL BARTH ON AGENCY IN DYING

In the above account, I have attempted to give a thorough description of Barth's theological understanding of human dying. In concluding this chapter, I will briefly describe the attitude or posture that Barth believes should characterize the believer's relationship with death and dying. In particular, our interest lies in the question of whether, and to what degree, Barth believes that we ought to be actively involved in the manner of our dying or whether one's relationship with one's death ought to be passively endured.

Barth most directly addresses this question in §56, titled "Freedom in Limitation." The section begins with this affirmation: "God the Creator wills and claims the man who belongs to Him, is united to his fellow-man and under obligation to affirm his own life and that of others, with the special intention indicated by the limit of time, vocation, and honour which He has already set him as his Creator and Lord" (*CD* III.4, 565). This means that every aspect of human existence (i.e., one's vertical relation to God, one's horizontal relations with neighbors, and one's integral self-relation as a psychosomatic unity) stands under various limits of which Barth names "time, vocation, and honour." How ought we to relate to each of these "limits"?

To answer the question, a word about Barth's ethics is in order.[30] Barth's has been called a "divine command" ethic, but we must immediately distinguish what Barth means by "command of God" (*CD* II.2, 516) from what is usually understood by that term. The divine command, rather than taking the form of universally applicable rules or ethical principles, is for Barth something that is received from God in the moment of ethical responsibility. Barth was not advocating an ethical mysticism of direct divine illumination or self-confident reliance on "leadings" from the Spirit. In the simplest terms, for Barth the divine command is a person, Jesus Christ.[31] Jesus Christ is the "indicative" statement of God concerning humankind, which becomes an "imperative" for human action. "What is the command of God? It is the authentic interpretation in the imperative mood of man's being and nature by its Creator and Lord" secured and revealed in Jesus Christ (*CD* III.4, 568).

This does not mean that the life and words of Jesus Christ become the moral standard according to which the Christian ought to live, at least not directly. There are important differences between Jesus and us that must be acknowledged and that prohibit his life from being an ethical template for our own. What the responsible moral agent seeks, according to Barth's version of the divine command, is a creaturely and faithful "correspondence" with the basic reality of the gospel revealed in Jesus Christ. In Barth's words, "when God meets man as his Commander, the result is that man must recognize his own nature and being in its correspondence to the command of God" (*CD* III.4, 567).

What does "correspondence" mean with respect to the temporal limitation of human life, which comes to us all through death? According to Barth, "the unique opportunity . . . is simply human life in its limitation by birth and death. And the imperative of the command, to the extent that its target is the freedom of man within the limitation of his nature and being, is simply that this unique opportunity must be *apprehended, grasped* and *used* by man. . . . All other limitations and determinations of human nature and being are in some way enclosed in and contained by this first one. It represents all the others" (*CD* III.4, 569). What I take this quotation to be suggesting is the following: death represents the "limitedness" of human life (of which temporal limitation is only one type). The posture toward this limitedness, which corresponds to the reality given to us in Jesus Christ, is not rebellion or resentment but rather affirmation, trust, and gratitude. These responses grow out of an appreciation of the once-and-for-all nature of human life: each and every life is a unique and singular opportunity. Thus, for Barth, "when God distinguishes and therefore limits, there can be no talk of a curtailment or impoverishment or deprivation of the one thus limited. His very limiting is His definite, concrete and specific affirmation. The man who is limited by Him is the man who is loved by Him. Rather than tolerating our limitation with a sigh, we have every reason to take it seriously, to affirm it, to accept it, and praise God for the fact that in it we are what we are and not something else" (*CD* III.4, 568).

The ethical question, then, becomes, am I at this moment "seizing or neglecting the unique opportunity" presented to me at this time? Barth offers several "criteria" of obedience in limited time: (a) Our limited time is treated with "the greatest possible openness and yet also the greatest possible resolution" (*CD* III.4, 585), by which Barth means that we must be open to learning from others who come before us or with whom we are in community, but ultimately we must resolve on obedience individually ("undoubtedly an act in isolation," *CD* III.4, 586) a resolution that takes the character of risk. (b) To seize one's unique opportunity, one must "know how to make time and to take time," by which Barth means that one cannot see life as a spectator but must be present and attentive to the task at hand. One cannot waste time or eschew the responsibility to choose but must take part wholeheartedly in that which claims her. (c) The one who seizes her unique opportunity "always remembers that [s]he will die and yet never fears death" (*CD* III.4, 588). To fail to really recognize that one day one will die is to "fail to be what we really are" and to become a stranger to oneself. "That we must and shall die . . . has to be accepted as a familiar element in our life. . . . If we do not consider that we shall die; if we do not press on from this truth to the required openness and resolution; if we do not let it forbid us to lose time and command us to make time for ourselves, then we are not genuinely and properly what we are" (*CD* III.4, 589).

But wait. Are we not here in danger of glorifying death? Barth would surely reply in the negative. For Barth, life is always a gift that commands "respect." Indeed, it is a bedrock truth that, because human life is directly dependent on the initiative and address of the Creator God, "man's creaturely existence as such is not his property; it is a loan" (*CD* III.4, 327) that is to be received and protected as such. Barth speaks affirmatively of medicine and the desire to mitigate sickness through the medical art. "The realm of death which afflicts man in the form of sickness . . . is opposed to His good will as Creator and has existence and power only under His mighty No. To capitulate before it, to allow it to take its course, can never be obedience but only disobedience towards God. In harmony with the will of God, what humans ought to will in face of this whole realm on the left hand, and therefore in face of sickness, can only be final resistance. . . . Those who take up this struggle obediently are already healthy in the fact that they do so, and theirs is no empty desire when they will to maintain or regain their health" (*CD* III.4, 366–69). The respect for life, however, does not mean its absolute and unqualified preservation and prolongation:

> Is it really true that the command of God in all cases and circumstances contains the imperative that man should will to live? Must not this imperative in some cases at least be formulated in what is from the literal standpoint a very paradoxical sense if it is really to be understood as the command of God? Understood in its most literal sense, it is hardly an unconditional and absolutely valid imperative which as such has necessarily to be included in every form of the divine command. Precisely as the command of God, does it not have a restricted validity, since the God who commands is not only the Lord of life but also the Lord of death? Is it really so unthinkable that, when his command summons man to freedom before Him and fellowship with his fellow-men, it might include a very different imperative, or *this imperative in its most paradoxical formulation*, to the effect that man should not will to live unconditionally, to spare his life, to preserve it from death, but that he should rather will to stake and surrender it, and perhaps be prepared to die? (*CD* III.4, 334–35)

Barth does not here, nor does he ever, advocate the taking of one's life through suicide, PAS, or euthanasia. Rather, he opens up space for a form of acceptance of death as a paradoxical expression of the command of God. We must emphasize that this acceptance of death is not the opposite of respect for life. According to Barth, respect for life is an unconditional element of the divine command. There are no "exceptions."[32] What respect for life might entail, however, cannot be wholly determined a priori in a way that precludes the responsibility of the moral agent before God. Barth is saying that in light of God's lordship over life *and death* and in light of all that has been said above about the goodness of creaturely finitude, there is a way in which the acceptance of death witnesses to the gospel truth of human dependence on and trust in God and, as such, actually affirms and respects precisely the form of life (i.e., limited, singular, dependent) that we actually have from God. This "respects life" more than a desperate, autonomous grasping after life, which can reduce the thing sought to "bare" life.

The answer to the question of the mode of agency vis-à-vis death and dying which corresponds with the divine command—that is, with Jesus Christ—can be found here. In learning to see death as a God-given boundary—while simultaneously affirming life as a God-given gift—human beings learn what it means to be (actually) the finite, dependent creatures we are (ultimately). Barth's entire theological anthropology, we might say, is written to drive home the point that the moral life of the human being exists largely in learning to be finite, to accept the fundamentally limited nature of the human condition. To do so, one must learn that the limits (e.g., of time, vocation, historical and geographic location, of interpersonal and relational dynamics, etc.) are not arbitrary but are given by God precisely in God's giving over to us our particular identity. What bounds us, then, at the limits is not nothing (and not "nothingness") but is God. This is the basis for a stance toward death that is basically receptive—while remaining responsible and attentive. This receptivity should perhaps be distinguished from pure "passivity," for it does require either a prior decision to be open and receptive, or a prior process of moral formation that results in such openness. The receptivity before death, which materially aligns with traditional proscriptions of deliberately ending a human life, flows from a different source and is animated by a different energy. It depends not so much on obedience to a rule or principle but rather flows from the freedom of living in active correspondence with the divine command, a freedom that, in this case, is the freedom to be patient and receptive and to find dignity and joy precisely in the giving over of the moment of death to the One who is Lord of death.

Autumn Alcott Ridenour elaborates on a Barthian understanding of agency in dying by exploring "the active and passive agency of Christ" in Barth's *Church Dogmatics*.[33] She notes,

> The twofold dynamic that entails Christ simultaneously serving as the eternal God who elects humanity and the elected human who responds to God reveals Christ's dual reality as both active and passive agent that involves the movement of giving and receiving. In Christ's divinity, he willingly or actively becomes human as the servant who goes into the far country. In Christ's humanity, he willingly responds to grace through receptive gratitude, humility, and obedience that ends in human exaltation and participation with God. . . . Here Barth reveals that to be human is to be a recipient or responsive agent to God's gracious summons by definition. The adequate human response to this divine invitation is a posture of prayerful response that enacts gratitude, humility, and obedience. Barth himself portrays the movement of divine giving and receiving, of action and passion, not only in Christ's person as a whole but particularly in the Gethsemane reality as an agent who moves from active to passive status.[34]

Ridenour places Barth in conversation with Canon W. H. Vanstone's *The Stature of Waiting* to illustrate the posture of passive agency. In it, Vanstone traces the narrative arc of the Gospel of Mark, highlighting the shift in verb mood from active to receptive after Jesus's prayer in the Garden of Gethsemane. Before this moment, Jesus was the subject of almost every verb; after this moment, he was the direct object of almost every verb. This is a posture that Christ freely enacted for the sake of love. According to Ridenour, "thus, even in Jesus's passion and his willingness to become object, he remains subject. In this way, the passion of Jesus remains both a divine and human act in his person."[35] Barth thereby highlights a notion of kenotic self-emptying, which expresses what humanity living in correspondence to God looks like.

Against the presumptions of the modern social imaginary that consider either autonomous control or individual authenticity the basis for human dignity, Jesus demonstrates that a special type of human dignity is actually revealed precisely in this "giving over." Such a posture is an expression of creaturely dependence before God, which is revealed to be true human correspondence to God in the action of Jesus Christ, the true human being. For the God revealed in scripture and in the incarnation is the "God who waits."[36] According to Ridenour, "Jesus's passive agency reveals the dignity of this world in that its value is worth waiting for, as seen through his endurance toward the cross. Vanstone argues that part of loving entails waiting—waiting on the other or waiting to receive the other."[37] For Vanstone, then, receptive agency, is not solely characteristic of human agency before God but is also mirrored in the Creator's mode of relation to the creature.

As with the "spirituality of martyrdom" in Roman Catholic moral theology, Barth's fundamental orientation of the human being in terms of "creaturely finitude" has the potential to radically alter many of our assumptions about human moral agency. In our own day in which we are increasingly likely to find ourselves the bearers of burdened agency at the end of life, the notion that the "handing over" of oneself to dependence—on God but also on family members or caretakers—is a very difficult task indeed. If the church were to reclaim the language of creatureliness, dependence, and finitude through its practices, then perhaps the Christian standpoint might generate new ways of engaging with medicine and other institutions at the end of life. To be sure, this does not provide robust action guides and therefore will not entirely relieve the sense of "burdening" I have described in this book. But it does have the potential to help Christians inhabit the institutions that exist with a renewed sense of hope and confidence—and thereby demonstrate to all people what it means to affirm the limited life we have.

FIVE

Stanley Hauerwas on Agency in Dying

Ethics of Dispossession

ETHICS FOR FINITE CREATURES

Burdened agency involves the sense that individuals are increasingly saddled with choices about how and when to die, while the frameworks of moral meaning and guidance that once guided such choices are largely falling away. This leaves dying as an increasingly individualistic and reflexive task. Stanley Hauerwas puts his finger on an important aspect of burdened agency. "What makes 'medical ethics' so difficult is the penchant of medical care to force decisions that seem to call into question aspects of our life that we assumed not to be matters of decision, e.g., should we provide medical care for children who are born with major disabilities?"[1] For the vast majority of persons in history, specifying the timing and nature of one's death has not been considered a matter of decision. To be sure, such things were suffered well or badly but were not typically "decided on."

In this chapter, I turn to the work of theologian and ethicist Stanley Hauerwas. Hauerwas's thought represents a culmination of the strands of theology explicated in chapters 3 and 4. Theologically trained at Yale Divinity School during the height of the Yale school and postliberal theology, Hauerwas has deeply Barthian sensibilities, especially with respect to the notion of "creaturely finitude."[2] This is especially evident in his emphasis on acceptance of tragedy and contingency in the moral life and in his nonfoundationalist theological and ethical methodology. Although he long ago moved to Duke University, some of Hauerwas's formative years were spent at the University of Notre Dame, where he regularly engaged colleagues about issues in Roman Catholic moral theology. His work is deeply resonant with the "spirituality of martyrdom" encouraged by thinkers like Servais Pinckaers and Karl Rahner. This aspect of his thought is especially evident in the way he weaves together insights about Christology and eschatology with reflections about virtue and character. In Hauerwas, this "spirituality of martyrdom" takes a pacifist key, yielding what I will call an "ethics of dispossession."

Hauerwas, then, provides the connection between theology and ecclesial practices. For it is through the church's formative liturgical practices that a new language is offered, shaping a new theological imagination that can help individual Christians approach their dying in ways that make the problem of burdened agency less acute.

A Few Notes on Hauerwas's Methodology

If Hauerwas is known for something apart from his unique accent and penchant for using colorful language, it is for giving constant attention to the interrelation between character (virtue), narrative (story), and community (ecclesial practices), especially as these coalesce around the theme of Christian nonviolence. Eschewing systematic coherence, in essay after essay Hauerwas elucidates an account of Christian ethics that refuses to begin from modern liberal presumptions about the nature of the self (as an individual, transcendental "I") and the self's way of knowing and choosing the good (in terms either of universal a priori "principles" or of a rational utilitarian calculus).[3]

In the introduction to *Truthfulness and Tragedy*, Hauerwas highlights three interrelated themes woven throughout the essays contained therein.

In fact, these themes play a prominent role in all of Hauerwas's work. I will therefore begin this chapter with a brief explanation of each of these themes to lay the groundwork for an account of Hauerwas's understanding of the relationship between death, dying, agency, and medicine. The basic themes are "(1) the nature of moral rationality and its significance for how theological ethics is conceived; (2) the interdependence of community and truthfulness; and (3) an understanding of the nature of Christian existence" as inescapably involving tragedy.[4] These three themes, taken together, demonstrate how deeply Hauerwas's thought is influenced by notions of creatureliness, finitude, and contingency.

The Nature of Moral Rationality:
Moving from Decisions to Descriptions

Hauerwas begins with an observation about the characteristic form of modern philosophy and ethics, whether in the mode of Kantianism, utilitarianism, or natural law: each of these seeks a foundation for moral rationality, which may elicit broad assent among those living in fragmented, pluralistic societies. To do so, modern ethics typically attempts to "free reason from the limits of particularistic communities." Hauerwas insists that such a project is futile. This conclusion, however, does not entail strong moral relativism. "There are 'criteria' of moral truthfulness, though such criteria can never be independent of a substantive narrative." Christian ethics, believes Hauerwas, "should begin with Christian convictions and how they shape our understanding of moral existence."[5] This means, of course, that one must temper one's desire for a universal ethical language (what Jeffrey Stout refers to as "moral Esperanto").[6] According to Hauerwas, "there is no such thing. . . . Ethics always requires an adjective or qualifier."[7]

To eschew moral Esperanto is to attempt Christian ethics in a manner that expresses one's nature as a finite, fallen, limited, and contingent creature. In other words, Hauerwas's form of ethics implies a certain theological anthropology. Hauerwas has clearly been influenced by Barth's paradoxical assertion that "ethics is sin."[8] As James Gustafson elaborates, "Ethics is sin if it assumes that a person, not God, has the prerogative of determining what is right and good."[9] This (sinful) goal is precisely that at which universalistic forms of ethics aim.

Hauerwas draws attention to one widespread implication of the presumption that ethics can proceed as if "from nowhere" — namely, an overemphasis on the discrete "act" or individual "decision" as the primary locus for moral evaluation. The resulting "quandary ethics" approach is especially pronounced within the realm of biomedical ethics, which often centers on the analysis of cases. "The very idea that ethics should be primarily concerned with 'quandaries' and the kind of decisions we ought to make about them," suggests Hauerwas, "reflects our current understanding of ourselves as a people without a history. 'Situations' are not 'out there' waiting to be seen but are created by the kind of people we are."[10] Elsewhere, Hauerwas elaborates, "the kind of agent we are and the kinds of institutions and practices in which we are involved determine the kinds of cases we confront. Situations are correlative of the ways we have learned to see, and seeing depends on the language we use and the expectations we have encouraged through our character and roles. . . . Ethical reflection, therefore, cannot concern itself exclusively with what we ought to do in certain dilemmas. It must be equally concerned about how we ought to see and understand what the dilemma is. We do not come to see just by looking; we must be trained to see rightly."[11]

Rather than focus on the moral justification of particular choices, therefore, Hauerwas prefers to focus on the process by which we come to understand and describe the situations that confront us and that create the context for our response. "The moral life is not first a life of choice—decision is not king—but is rather woven from the notions that we use to see and form the situations we confront. Moral life involves learning to see the world through an imaginative ordering of our basic symbols and notions."[12]

To illustrate Hauerwas's claim, it may be helpful at this point to consider a couple of examples. I will give one from the beginning of life and one from the end of life. Consider, for example, the issue of treating critically ill newborns. In the bioethics literature, this issue is almost always framed in terms of a "decision" to be made (recall, for example, the title of McCormick's influential essay "To Save or Let Die?"). This is, of course, understandable in light of the fact that bioethics journals are read by physicians who, as a matter of fact, have to make decisions.

Hauerwas, however, directs attention away from the moment of decision and toward the underlying assumptions about parenting that frame the dilemma itself. Many critically ill newborns face a high likelihood of suffering (though our ability to understand and predict the nature and intensity of such suffering remains limited) and a low likelihood of what we might label a "normal existence," characterized by participation in the full range of activities open to other children. In other words, such births preclude from the outset the achievement of two alleged parental duties: the prevention of suffering and the assurance of a happy or successful life. But should we assume these are the duties of parenthood? To be sure, we might judge those who fail to protect their child from exposure to certain harms (e.g., allowing a child to wander into a busy intersection) or who impede a child's development (e.g., through malnutrition or lack of education), but surely, it is unreasonable to expect a parent to ensure a child's happiness and prevent all suffering?

Apart from a critical evaluation of societal expectations of parental responsibility, we might fail to recognize the way "convictions like these reduce the options at birth to a perfect child or a dead child."[13] Rather, Hauerwas argues, "we cannot and should not raise our children as if they could be protected against suffering and death. I suspect that the greatest injustice in some of these neonatal cases is done because we have lost sight of the fact that we must learn to love and care for our children as being destined for death. . . . We should not under all conditions try to keep our children alive, but then neither should we kill some of our children because they do not conform to our ideal of 'the good life.'"[14] The point here is not to settle issues of neonatal intensive care and nontreatment but to point out that the very framing of the issue as a dilemma presupposes a community with certain linguistic practices (i.e., the meaning and expectations of "parenthood"). This obscures the fact that there are some for whom no such "decision" need be made at all, for whom the critical ethical question is how best to welcome the child who comes as a stranger, a stranger who is destined for a life that includes suffering and death.

Consider also Hauerwas's treatment of suicide and euthanasia. Hauerwas (with Richard Bondi) argues that the key issue in evaluating suicide and euthanasia is not the physical description of the act so much as the meaning it has in the larger social, moral, and cultural context. "Our notions, our descriptions, our very actions are held fast by stories, by the narratives that are our context for meaning. Ethics is the attempt to help us remember what kind of story sustains certain descriptions. It is, therefore, a discipline rather like history, in that we are forced to tell stories in order to capture our past, sustain our present, and give our future direction."[15] What is needed, then, is to get at the grammar of our moral notions.[16] According to Hauerwas and Bondi, "the story that should underlie the Christian understanding of suicide and euthanasia is not that of wider society."[17] The latter, for example, appeals to notions of "rights" (i.e., the right to die) grounded in the assumption that "we should be able to determine our lives, when our life will end, and what we shall do with it. But it is fundamental to the Christian manner that our lives are formed in terms not of what we will do with them, but of what God will do with our lives, both in our living and our dying. Life is not sacred as if we Christians had an interest in holding onto it to the last minute. Christians are a people who are formed ready to die for what they believe. . . . Life for us, therefore, is not an absolute, for that which we think gives our life form will not let us place unwarranted value on life itself."[18]

The problem with suicide and euthanasia is not simply that these acts contravene a natural desire to live but that they "tempt us to take on a story that will pervert our manner not only of dying but of living."[19] To speak of suicide and euthanasia in a manner schooled by the Christian story begins with an understanding of life as a gift—"not [a gift] like other gifts . . . not a property to possess . . . but a task to live out." In other words, life is "a gift of time enough for love"[20] of God and neighbor. This means that insofar as the Christian understands her life to be a responsibility to uphold the love and trust necessary to sustain community, she feels a duty to live and not die. (This, to forestall an obvious objection, does not imply that the duty to live is an absolute duty.)

For Hauerwas, then, "descriptions are everything,"[21] for prior to the moment of decision (both temporally and logically) lies the formation of the subject (including her disposition, habits, and social imaginary), which is itself unintelligible apart from her embeddedness in a narratively shaped linguistic community. Thus, Hauerwas traces the many connections between the stories we understand to frame our lives, the language that arises from these stories, and the way in which such language is institutionalized and reflected in our practical affairs, which in turn shape the character of the community itself.

The Interrelation of Community and Truthfulness

The second main theme of Hauerwas's work follows from the first. Ethics is a matter of learning and enacting a "language," but we must remember that language is a communal practice. A language cannot be merely private; it must exist among and between people—that is, in a community that shares a way of life that makes the use of language intelligible. Following Wittgenstein's insight that the meaning of language is found in its use, Hauerwas insists on a mutual connection between the truthfulness of a community's claims and the character of the community's way of life. On the one hand, the existence of a community is the necessary precondition for the existence of truthful speech. On the other hand, a "truthfulness is equally necessary for the building of noncoercive community."[22] For Hauerwas takes it as basic truth that precisely to the degree that community feels compelled to employ violence in the name of its convictions, those convictions are revealed to be inherently unstable because they are ultimately false.

What is perhaps Hauerwas's most programmatic account of the importance of "community," and by extension of "church," occurs in his book *The Peaceable Kingdom*. In that work, he reiterates his previous work on character and virtue, adding a further emphasis on moral formation. "We Christians ought not to search for the 'behavioral implications' of our beliefs. Our moral life is not comprised of beliefs plus decisions; our moral life is the process in which our convictions form our character to be truthful. . . . The Christian life is more a recognition and training of our senses and passions than a matter of choices and decisions."[23] This raises the question of how such formation is supposed to occur. We have already mentioned that moral formation is like learning a language. Alternatively, we might say that it is something like being apprenticed into a craft or trade.

Consider woodworking, for example. A master woodworker, when looking at a piece of oak or redwood, sees something essentially different from what I (lacking any woodworking experience whatsoever) might see. According to George Nakashima, "[each] flitch, each board, each plank can have only one ideal use. The woodworker, applying a thousand skills, must find that ideal use and then shape the wood to realize its true potentiality."[24] The master sees the "soul" of the tree, the way in which each and every facet of a piece of wood contributes to its suitability and potentiality to be used in a way that amplifies its beauty. Such vision, however, does not come "naturally." Nakashima was himself taught to see in such a way by a master in the art of Japanese woodworking while being held at an internment camp during World War II.[25]

This example highlights the necessarily interpersonal nature of formation—the inherent connection between community and tradition, between tradition and vision, between vision and character, and between character and action. Hauerwas notes, "We can only act within the world we can envision, and we can envision the world rightly only as we are trained to see. We do not come to see merely by looking, but must develop disciplined skills through initiation into that community that attempts to live faithful to the story of God."[26] For Hauerwas, then, the church is the community that carries forward—both articulated in words and embodied in practice—the story of God that makes possible a truthful seeing of the world. This forms the basis for Hauerwas's oft-quoted claim that the "first social ethical task of the church is to be the church" so that the world may know that it is "world."[27] For the church to "be the Church" involves becoming "a community that keeps alive the language of the faith through the liturgical, preaching and teaching offices of the community."[28] Living from a distinct story, with distinct linguistic practices and a distinct manner of life, the church constitutes an alternative to every other polis or civitas.

Here, a word about the "political" nature of Hauerwas's theological ethic may be in order, especially since (as we shall see in the next section) Hauerwas's evaluation of contemporary medicine is linked with his critique of modern political liberalism. Largely following from his claims that "the first task of the church is to be the church" and that "the church does not have, but *is* a social ethic," Hauerwas has been repeatedly charged with advocating a "sectarian" ethic of "withdrawal" from the various institutions of public life. As a result, it is sometimes claimed that Hauerwas and other "Neo-Anabaptists" are apolitical or quietistic. In reality, the opposite is the case. In almost every essay, Hauerwas is making a political argument. Hauerwas's answer to such claims is that "any theology reflects a politics, whether that politics is acknowledged or not. The crucial question is: what *kind* of politics is theologically assumed?"[29]

The sectarian charge typically relies on a particularly narrow definition of politics as involving the task to secure justice or common interest through the apparatus of the liberal democratic state. Hauerwas notes that he was trained in the tradition of Christian social ethics, which, following Rauschenbusch and Reinhold Niebuhr, took for granted the fact that "democratic politics was normative for Christians" and that Christians have a fundamental responsibility to participate in the structures of power as they exist. This assumption, however, was challenged — and ultimately dismantled — through his engagement with John Howard Yoder. Already before encountering Yoder, Hauerwas had begun to drive a wedge between democratic practices and liberal political and economic theory, the latter he sees as problematically undermining the social virtues necessary to sustain the former.[30] From Yoder, Hauerwas learned to resist "any politics that portrays the church as apolitical in a manner that leaves the formation of the body to the state." In contrast, Yoder supplied Hauerwas with an understanding of the church as "a political space in its own right," which need not overly concern itself with the governing structures of the land. According to Yoder, to ask "what is the best form of government?" is itself a Constantinian question insofar as it "presupposes that the one asking the question is in an 'established' social posture that presumes a position of power."[31] This is not the position that we can or should expect those within the church of Jesus Christ to hold.

What is it in particular that Hauerwas finds so corrosive about liberalism? For one, Hauerwas contends, "the liberal commitment to the freedom of the individual does not provide an ethos sufficient for the nurturing of morally truthful lives."[32] There is, according to Hauerwas, a "peculiar form of self-deception at the heart of the modern project." For the liberal commitment to creating free individuals implies that "you should have no story except the story you have chosen when you had no story." But who among us, in a liberal society, is truly able to "choose the story that we should have no story except the story we have chosen from the position where we allegedly had no story"?[33]

In the next section, we will return to this critique to demonstrate how, in Hauerwas's estimation, the liberal commitment to autonomy and freedom (of a certain sort) underlies the practices of modern medicine in a way that makes it difficult to achieve a good death. For now, let me simply draw attention to one further aspect of Hauerwas's critique of liberalism that will also introduce the third major theme in Hauerwas's theological ethics.

The Tragic Character of Human Existence

For Hauerwas, both the modern liberal search for a universal foundation for ethics and the commitment to "freedom of the individual" are symptoms of a deep fear and denial of the tragic character of human existence, especially as this relates to the moral life. Because Hauerwas believes that a central criterion of the truthfulness of any narrative is that it "give[s] us the means to accept the tragic without succumbing to self-deceiving explanations," he drives home his critique of liberalism at precisely this point.[34]

What does Hauerwas mean by tragedy? It is not the same as suffering. Tragedy involves suffering, but there are forms of suffering that are not inherently tragic. Consider, for example, a day in the life of a competitive runner: she wakes early (forgoing sleep), eats meticulously (forgoing even the smallest of indulgences), trains rigorously multiple times per day (experiencing pain and physical exhaustion in the process), often leaving little to no time for social life and friendship. Subordinated and incorporated as they are within a life project that gives them meaning, these difficulties are not tragic: they are, rather, the fruit and the evidence of the pursuit of a worthy human goal.

One form of tragic suffering follows from our having and keeping substantive moral commitments that cannot intrinsically be incorporated into a larger project (like the one mentioned in the previous paragraph). The obvious example in this case is the suffering of the Christian (or religious) martyr, but importantly, suffering can also redound to others as a result of our moral convictions. Hauerwas recognizes, for example, that a commitment to nonviolence will at times involve the tragic, and otherwise preventable, suffering of innocent people. Similarly, in medicine, the physician's covenantal relationship to the individual patient constrains the pursuit of certain potential goods that would require undermining her commitment to her patient (e.g., in the conflict between clinical research and medical care).

Although not always recognized, tragedy is an enduring feature of the moral life as such. Attention to tragedy, however, is especially important in understanding the vocation of medicine. Medicine is a "tragic profession"[35] because of the very nature of the endeavor to care for another person under the conditions of finitude and fallenness.[36] For example, we may understand fairly well the pathology and disease process of sepsis, but we cannot infallibly predict its onset or the particular patient's reaction to a chosen treatment.

Moreover, in medicine, one is sometimes confronted with apparently pointless suffering that cannot be cured. Of course, it is not that medicine is somehow "more tragic" than other aspects of our lives, but "its practice manifests and embodies more intensely the tragic nature of our existence."[37]

In light of these three key themes in Hauerwas's approach to ethics (narrative, community, and tragedy), let us now turn to a broader discussion of his evaluation of modern medical practice. Medicine nourished by the narratives of liberal modernity, according to Hauerwas, fails to recognize the inevitability of tragedy and death. The sad result is that such medicine often serves to exacerbate and intensify the sense of tragedy at the end of life.

HAUERWAS'S UNDERSTANDING OF MODERN MEDICINE

The Story Most of Us Live By

As we have seen, in Hauerwas's telling, "the project of modernity was to produce people who believe they should have no story except the story they choose when they have no story. Such a story is called the story of freedom and is assumed to be irreversibly institutionalized economically as market capitalism and politically as democracy."[38] Hauerwas is here pulling together strands from various Enlightenment thinkers but especially from the social contract tradition of political thought. Social contract theories attempt to articulate the fundamental principles that unite individuals into a society. Each of these theories imagines the atomized "individual" as the fundamental unit of society, existing in some sense prior to the social bonds that exist between persons—though theorists disagree about the nature of this hypothetical individual, whether he (it's almost always "he") is defined by his pursuit of self-interest and security (Hobbes), his possession of natural rights (Locke), or freedom of will (Rousseau). What these theories hold in common can be seen especially in John Rawls's version of the social contract that imagines individuals deciding about the fundamental rules of society from an "original position" behind a "veil of ignorance" regarding the particularities that will define each of them once the rules have been agreed on.[39] The view of the individual here is what Michael Sandel famously referred to as the myth of the "unencumbered self."[40] When human beings are imagined in this way, as basically "bundles of rights and preferences,"[41] then freedom is seen as the ability to choose between competing options.

Such theories, according to Hauerwas, "entail a moral psychology that suggests if an agent is to be free she must be capable of 'standing back' from her own action so that she will not be fated by the past."[42] The liberal understanding of the autonomy of the individual therefore requires the eradication of tragedy from our sense of human agency (a point to which we will return below). Echoing Kant, Hauerwas ironically claims, "Chance or fate to the modern ethicist represents an irrational surd. We all know that morality must have to do only with those matters that we can do something about. Control, not chance, is the hallmark of the moral man."[43]

There is a second version of the liberal story of the self that Hauerwas sometimes tells. We might call this version the Hobbesian version, over against the Kantian/Rawlsian picture just described. According to the Hobbesian story, "'liberalism' names those societies wherein it is presupposed that the only thing people have in common is their fear of death, despite the fact that they share no common understanding of death. So, liberalism is that cluster of theories about society that are based on the presumption that we must finally each die alone."[44] Hobbes's account assumes that the fear of death and the desire for security are the driving motives behind social interactions. This fear of death is manifested politically in the authority granted to the state to wage wars (internationally) and enforce laws (domestically), but we can also see it in the extraordinary authority granted to the institutions of modern medicine and public health.

The Medicine We Desire, the Medicine We Deserve

Given what has been said thus far, it would not be difficult to conclude that Hauerwas is "anti-medicine" or that he, in some sense, blames the medical profession for society's woes. In fact, nothing could be further from the truth. Hauerwas considers it extraordinary that a group of people exists whose fundamental professional responsibility is to keep company with the sick. We should not forget the fact that those who are sick experience pain and suffering, which by its very nature threatens to bring about radical isolation. Physicians, whose fundamental responsibility, according to Hauerwas, is to care for patients even when they cannot cure them, "are the bridge between the world of the ill and the healthy."[45] This responsibility is what makes medicine a moral art.

Granted, we must at once note that the practice of medicine does not occur in a vacuum. It may be a substantive moral practice in its own right, but like all institutions, it is influenced by the broader society within which it is practiced. In fact, medicine may be particularly susceptible to such influence, for the commitment to be present with those who suffer illness is incredibly difficult to uphold, argues Hauerwas, if it is not continually sustained by the practices of a substantive moral community.

Medicine cannot help but become distorted when set in the context of a culture that prizes freedom and autonomy above all else. If this occurs (and Hauerwas argues that it has), we should not rush to blame the medical establishment. We get "precisely the kind of medicine we deserve."[46] We have noted in previous chapters how various technological developments and institutional arrangements drive a type of medicine that places concrete decisions about the nature and timing of death in the hands of individuals who do not typically know how to bear their agency well. What has not been sufficiently recognized is the fact that burdened agency, though often unwanted at the point of deciding, is largely a self-induced problem. The expectations placed on medicine by patients explain much of our current moral situation. If the medicine we have "reflects who we are, what we want, and what we fear" and "the way we think about death,"[47] then "the fault lies with those of us who pretentiously place undue expectations on medicine in the hope of finding an earthly remedy to our death."[48] For "if we share anything as a people, it is that death ought to be avoided in the hope we can finally get out of life alive."[49]

Medicine and the Project of Anthropodicy

Why, according to Hauerwas, do we burden medicine with such overblown expectations? Although there are probably many reasons for this, the main reason is that medicine has become the primary way of dealing with the problem of evil in a pluralistic, secular, and therapeutic culture. "Theodicy," or the defense of God in light of the problem of evil, has long been a preoccupation of Christian theologians and philosophers. As scientific and technological capacity increased the scope of human power and the God of Abraham, Isaac, Jacob, and Jesus is replaced by the God of Deism, theodicy gives way to anthropodicy. What needs to be justified in light of suffering is not God but humankind.

The suffering that is most problematic is the suffering we assume to be under our control. Natural disasters, of course, do not seem to qualify, but "sickness is quite another matter. . . . Sickness challenges our most cherished presumption that we are or at least can be in control of our existence."[50] Medicine, then, becomes one of the primary institutions—if not *the* primary institution—through which anthropodicy is channeled. In this context, "can" implies "ought," and therapeutic medical intervention becomes completely self-justifying. To the degree that medicine is loaded with such expectations, adequate "medical care" becomes equated with being able to bring about a "cure." The result is a distortion of medicine's primary calling, which is presence in the face of suffering. Of course, caring and curing are not mutually exclusive acts, and there are times (many, in fact) when the most caring thing a physician can do is help a patient achieve real healing. However, when the imperative to "cure" occludes a deeper responsibility to care, medicine becomes fundamentally distorted. As a result, those who cannot be cured tend to be isolated by the medicine that should, in principle, stand as a bridge between the worlds of the sick and the well. Additionally, when medicine is equated with curing, other goals of care (e.g., assisting the process of coping with incurable illness) are neglected. Not only that, but the equation of medicine with curing encourages physicians to view death as a "failure." Of course, there may be instances of death that result from medical failures (e.g., death as a result of negligence or ineptitude), but death as such is not a medical failure; it is a biological inevitability. To treat it as a failure of medicine is to burden medical professionals and patients alike with unrealistic, counterproductive, and sometimes harmful expectations.

Killing Compassion

Most of us would agree that one should prevent suffering when possible. And yet, there are unintended consequences that arise from making this a universal principle of medicine. For one, it virtually guarantees the perpetual expansion of technological interventions. For those who may have anxieties about the implementation or development of particular technologies, it is very hard to argue against the appeals to compassion and the prevention of suffering. Ironically, Hauerwas suggests, the very desire to eliminate suffering may have, if we are not careful, the effect of causing new, unintended forms of suffering. So, for example, an early essay of Hauerwas's explores the overtreatment of critically ill neonates, cautioning against a "mercy grown overwhelming by technology."[51] Elsewhere, Hauerwas declaims "the increasing subjection of our lives to a technology grown cruel by its Promethean pretensions."[52]

It is not the use of technology per se that is problematic. Neither is Hauerwas opposed to relief of suffering. But compassion can become an overriding virtue in a society that is unable to acknowledge the tragic nature of human existence. Moreover, it makes perfect sense that compassion has achieved self-validating status to those of us who live in liberal societies. For we are aware of our deep fragmentation regarding ultimate ends and objects of morality and have a political system that claims agnosticism regarding such matters. Compassion, however, as Oliver O'Donovan has noted, is "a virtue of motivation rather than reasoning," which "presupposes that an answer has already been found to the question 'what needs to be done?'"[53]

Hauerwas, ever the contrarian, challenges the idea that compassion is an adequate and desirable guiding norm for social practices. One clue that compassion is not morally adequate lies in the way our society treats the mentally handicapped. We rightly lament the suffering that accompanies certain genetic disorders and cognitive disabilities, and we desire to minimize their impact. (Although, to be sure, it is easy to overestimate the amount of "suffering" that is experienced by someone with, for example, Down syndrome or autism spectrum disorder.) Such cognitive disabilities, however, are not like many other "diseases," for to "cure" the disability would have the effect of eradicating the very person herself. Of course, there is no widespread campaign for the practice of involuntary euthanasia of persons with cognitive disabilities.[54] There are, however, subtle pressures that are sometimes present in medical encounters that may dissuade people, for example, from bringing a pregnancy to term once a prenatal diagnosis of Down syndrome has been made. When, as in cases like these, we seek to eliminate the one who suffers in the name of the elimination of suffering, "compassion literally becomes a killer."[55]

Examples of such "killing compassion" are not limited to questions of abortion but also apply to physician-assisted suicide and euthanasia.[56] It is no coincidence that such actions are often referred to as "mercy killings." The motivation of relief of suffering is constituent in the notion of euthanasia, as defined, for example, by both the Roman Catholic Church's Congregation of the Doctrine of Faith and major professional codes of ethics.

There are, however, problematic assumptions at play in such efforts. It will be important to outline such assumptions and name what is problematic about them, but if we are to follow Hauerwas, we must first attend to the particularities of the Christian narrative of suffering and death. For ethics, as Hauerwas demonstrates, must always begin in medias res. There is no neutral and nonhistorical starting point from which we could adjudicate such issues in the abstract. The way forward, if there is one, involves a very particular kind of casuistry, according to which "a tradition tests whether its practices are consistent (that is, truthful) or inconsistent in the light of its basic habits and convictions or whether these convictions require new practices and behavior."[57] These convictions, however, are not freestanding "ideas" or "beliefs," which may be detached from the formation of a particular community over time as its members try to live in light of "the narrative that has bound [their] lives" together.[58]

In the following section, we will outline some of the elements of the Christian narrative, as articulated by Hauerwas, which are pertinent to our understanding of agency in dying and of the relationship between the church and individual Christians in approaching end-of-life issues. In doing so, we will focus on Hauerwas's remarks on the nature and role of suffering in the Christian life and on the nature and meaning of Christ's death in particular, as well as the virtues needed to die well.

DEATH, SUFFERING, AND THE CHRISTIAN STORY

Dying for the Right Thing

How are Christians to understand death and suffering? What meaning can they find in the face of these things that will enable them to go on? Hauerwas is not a systematic theologian, so we should not expect anything so comprehensive as a "theology of death" from him. Additionally, given his critical comments regarding the project of theodicy, Hauerwas will nowhere offer an "explanation" of death that seeks to remove its offense. Nevertheless, the issues he writes about often require him to explicate aspects of the Christian narrative that bear on our understanding of death. Moreover, he does at times make more general observations about the way the Christian tradition has understood human mortality in light of its basic story.

For example, in an early essay titled, "The Ethics of Death: Letting Die or Putting to Death?" Hauerwas acknowledges the prevalence of "moral reflection about death in terms of such issues as euthanasia and suicide" but notes "there has been little sustained ethical reflection on death as a necessary aspect of our life project; such reflection is necessary if we are to be able to deal with death in its everyday form."[59] According to Hauerwas, one finds an ambiguous posture toward death in scripture. Death "is at once seen as an enemy yet accepted as necessary and natural aspect of our lives." This ambivalence "sets the boundaries for any general discussion of death."[60] On the one hand, the "message of the gospel does not remove the fact of our death" but rather "teaches us the appropriate kind of fear of death." In general, death is to be avoided and is rightly feared. We cannot blithely claim that death is our friend, that it is good and welcome. Such platitudes betray a denial of tragedy. Although death is to be feared, however, "the proper fear of death can be perverted, especially if it takes the form of the ideology of the absoluteness of life."[61] Hauerwas is critical of appeals to the "sanctity of life" when such appeals imply that a Christian believes that life is an end in itself. "No one lives just to live." Life is about more than mere biological functioning. The purposes of the Christian life are "determined by the purposes of God as manifest in the history of Israel and Jesus's cross and resurrection."[62]

The subordination of both life and death to a higher spiritual good is related to one of the guiding images in Hauerwas's work: that the Christian life is one of witness (*marturios*).[63] The primary goal of Christian life is not to make the world better but to bear witness to the God who saved Israel from slavery and who raised Jesus from the dead. In bearing this witness, the church shows the world what it means to be "world," which is to say, what it means to be ignorant and opposed to the truth of the gospel. The key insight is that Christian life has a performative and communicative aspect: the way of life of a Christian is to convey something about the narrative she takes to be true. But as the example of the martyrs makes vivid, this performative element can, and often is, as important in the way one dies as in the way one lives. The name "martyr" (witness) is given to those Christians who meet their death faithfully rather than capitulate to a false story. This is the goal of every Christian. Thus, according to Hauerwas, Christians are primarily concerned not with extending life but with dying "for the right thing." Christians should not speak of "sanctity of life" in a way that implies that they believe "there is nothing in life worth dying for."[64] Rightly understood, "dying is not the tragedy but, from our point of view, dying for the wrong thing."[65] Indeed, one of the things that makes Christians distinctive is their recognition "that their deaths are not an unmitigated disaster," for "service to one another is more important than life itself."[66] Because of this, Christians, like the martyrs, should be marked by a "peculiar readiness to die."[67]

Hauerwas here echoes the "spirituality of martyrdom" elaborated in the conclusion to chapter 3. There, we emphasized the concept of martyrdom as "obedience unto death," expressed through a particular mode of agency we called "submissive receptivity." Hauerwas here draws the connection between the martyr's mode of agency and her view of death as neither a good thing in itself nor an absolute evil. As Pinckaers noted, what was central to martyrs' spirituality was the way that their suffering was related to the suffering of Jesus Christ. Their suffering mirrored Christ's kenotic, self-emptying love. Hauerwas's understanding of martyrdom is likewise illuminated through his Christology—for Christology provides the key for understanding the martyr as the one whose faithfulness is expressed through the ultimate act of dispossession. In the following section, we will elaborate the nature of this Christ-shaped "ethic of dispossession."

Hauerwas's Kenotic Christology

As mentioned, to treat death as an absolute and utter evil is not a scriptural position. This, however, is not a conclusion reached through general observation but one that follows from the Christian narrative and especially the life, death, and resurrection of Jesus Christ. This brings up the centrality of Christology to Hauerwas's understanding of both creation and ethics. Although Hauerwas is not particularly known for attention to Christology,

Richard Hays is correct in remarking that an emphasis on the centrality of Jesus Christ is "the deepest theme in [Hauerwas's] work, the consistent thread running through all his thought."[68]

One essay in particular is important for understanding how Christology informs Hauerwas's understanding of suffering and death, for it explains how the nature of the Kingdom, revealed in Jesus Christ, is one of dispossession and patience that makes it possible to "live out of control." "Jesus: The Presence of the Peaceable Kingdom" is the central chapter in arguably one of the central books in Hauerwas's corpus.[69] In this chapter, Hauerwas argues that essential to understanding the scriptural portrayal of Jesus is the theme of *imitatio Dei*, for "the very heart of following the way of God's kingdom involves nothing less than learning to be like God" (75). Hauerwas notes that the command to "be perfect, as your heavenly Father is perfect" (Matt 5:48) is not a command that Jesus invented but draws on "the long habits of thought developed in Israel through her experience with the Lord" (76). Israel understood its history in terms of God's saving acts toward the people of God and their responsiveness to those acts. This responsiveness is constitutive of Israel's identity. "Israel is Israel . . . just to the extent that she 'remembers' the 'way of the Lord,' for by that remembering she in fact imitates God" (77). As this quotation indicates (in a way that should bring to mind Barth's divine command ethic), "imitation" here indicates less a direct equality of action (as if that were possible) than a correspondence of action. The people of God reflect God's character by remembering and responding in light of God's prior action. This mode of imitation was a communal act, incumbent on every Israelite but embodied in the major offices of prophet, priest, and king.

According to Hauerwas, the earliest Christians understood Jesus as the "continuation of Israel's vocation to imitate God and thus in a decisive way to depict God's kingdom for the world" (78). This fact provides the crucial context for understanding the significance of the wilderness temptations. Will Jesus capitulate to "Israel's perennial desire for a certainty of her own choosing" by asserting himself as the prophet who, like Moses, can turn stone into bread? Will Jesus grasp at a worldly form of kingship by accepting dominion over the nations? Will Jesus twist the role of priest by forcing "God's hand by being the sacrifice that God cannot refuse" (79)? In each of these cases, Jesus is tempted by a form of *imitatio Dei*, which is distorted to the degree that it attempts to control one's destiny rather than trust and respond to the God who has already proved trustworthy. Jesus's response to such temptations, however, demonstrates that true "imitation" of God comes by way of renunciation—especially the renunciation of (a certain sort of) power. "Jesus's whole life . . . is a life of power that is possible only for one possessed by the power of God. But such a power, exactly because it is a genuine and truthful power, does not serve by forcing itself on others" (80–81). In fact, "the form of power which results from our being dispossessed of the powers currently holding our lives can come only as we freely give up those things and goods that possess us. But we do not dispossess ourselves just by our willing, but by being offered a way of selfless power" (81). This is precisely what Jesus models and offers in the cross.

> In Jesus' life we cannot help but see God's way with Israel and Israel's subsequent understanding of what it means to be God's beloved. For God does not impose his will upon her. Rather he calls her time and time again to his way, to be faithful to the covenant, but always gives Israel the possibility of disobedience. It is thus in the cross that Christians see the climax of God's way with the world. In his cross we see decisively the one who, being all-powerful, becomes vulnerable even to being a victim of our refusal to accept his lordship. (81)

The cross, then, reveals the nature of the kingdom.[70] It is an apocalyptic in-breaking of the kingdom, which gives Christians eyes "to see the world . . . eschatologically" (82). The cross, however, is not separable and distinct from Jesus's life but is its culmination and fullest expression. Jesus is the *autobasileia*, the Kingdom Himself, in life *and* in death. One of the hallmarks of the kingdom, as revealed in the cross, is a trusting and faithful willingness to be dispossessed of all one has. This is not, Hauerwas cautions, to say that the cross stands as a "general symbol of the moral significance of self-sacrifice." Rather, "the cross is Jesus's ultimate dispossession through which God has conquered the powers of this world. The cross is not just a symbol of God's kingdom; *it is* that kingdom come."[71]

The Ethics of Dispossession

For Hauerwas, the Christian life is a matter of learning to let one's life be conformed to the Kingdom, which means that "discipleship is quite simply extended training in being dispossessed" (86). Although this may entail a willingness to part with material possessions, Hauerwas is not interested in advocating material poverty. What we are in most need of being dispossessed of is not our "things" but our compulsive need to be in control. It is this need that causes us to turn to violence and coercion—the very principalities and powers over which Jesus triumphed in the cross—to secure our significance and safety. Because Christ's victory over the powers has been affirmed and vindicated in the resurrection, Christians have an eschatological confidence and hope that ultimate victory does not and cannot depend on their own efforts. Therefore, "we can rest in God because we are no longer driven by the assumption that we must be in control of history, that it is up to us to make things come out right" (87). Not only are Christians dispossessed of control because of the eschatological victory of Christ; they are also dispossessed of control by the fact that they live as a forgiven people. The acceptance of forgiveness necessarily requires one to acknowledge one's guilt, to eschew self-justification, and to entrust oneself to another.

The "essential link," according to Hauerwas, between the acceptance of forgiveness and the ability to live as a peaceable people, is the way in which the dispossession of control entailed in forgiveness provides a way to accept our stories. For "when we exist as a forgiven people we are able to be at peace with our histories, so that now God's life determines our whole way of being—our character. We no longer need to deny our past, or tell ourselves false stories, as now we can accept what we have been without the knowledge of our sin destroying us" (89). Forgiveness invites us to make our lives our own by locating them within a broader story of Jesus's life, death, and resurrection, and the corresponding story of the worshipping community's response to this reality.

The ethical correlative of learning to live out of control is acquiring the "grace of doing nothing" (135).[72] For Hauerwas, "doing nothing" will at times be the only faithful response available to the Christian who refuses to use violent or coercive means to ensure a propitious outcome. "Doing nothing," however, is not to be equated with mere passivity. The Christian inactivity advocated by Hauerwas is a prophetic resistance to the powers, which relies for its coherence on substantive theological commitments. As becomes clear to anyone acquainted with Hauerwas's works, his is paradoxically an active inactivity, a pugnacious peaceableness, a combative nonviolent witness. For such a posture to be sustained, argues Hauerwas, requires a spirituality that acknowledges the tragic character of Christian existence but also acknowledges the ultimate victory of Christ. Such a posture does not typically arise on its own but must be cultivated. Especially important is the cultivation of the virtues of hope and patience:

> Christians must acquire a spirituality which will make them capable of being faithful in the face of the inexorable tragedies their convictions entail. A spirituality that acknowledges the tragic is one that is schooled in patience. As H. Richard Niebuhr suggested, our unwillingness to employ violence in order to make the world "better" means that we must often learn to wait. Yet such waiting must resist the temptation to cynicism, conservatism, or false utopianism that assumes the process of history will result in "everything coming out all right." For Christians hope not in "the processes of history," but in the God whom we believe has already determined the end of history in the cross and resurrection of Jesus Christ. Without such a declaration, patience in the face of the tragic could as easily be but a stoic acquiescence to fate. (145)

To recap: Hauerwas's *theologia crucis* gives rise to an ethic of dispossession—especially "being dispossessed of the illusion of security and power that is the breeding ground of our violence" (148).[73] In much of his work, Hauerwas seeks to demonstrate how dispossession is a necessary precondition for living a life that is faithful to the gospel, especially in its commitment to nonviolence. The moral implications of dispossession, however, go beyond the issue of nonviolence.[74] I suggest that "dispossession" can be a rich source of theological reflection for considering the ethics of death and dying. For what is dying but a process of gradual and, eventually, total dispossession? The loss of physical strength and coordination as well as mental and cognitive capacity are clear examples of this. Even more, studies show that what people fear most of all in advanced old age and at the end of life is not pain and suffering but loss of control. The fear of dying is in actuality a fear of being dispossessed. Surely, such dispossession is inevitably difficult and unpleasant and, at times, harrowing and dreadful. Who can better face such a prospect than the Christian who has already undergone a lifelong training in dispossession? Of course, this is true only to the degree that Christians have been shaped by the story of Christ's cross (which dispossesses us of the fallen and violent principalities and powers) and Christ's resurrection (which dispossesses us of the need to control the course of history) rather than the narratives of liberal modernity (which makes self-possession essential to personhood and dignity).

CONCLUSION: LESSONS FROM L'ARCHE FOR CHRISTIAN AGENCY IN DYING

This chapter has been building toward the Christological "ethic of dispossession" that unites the theological strands presented in the previous two chapters (i.e., the spirituality of martyrdom and the acceptance of creaturely finitude). We have all along been looking to articulate the Christian standpoint in terms that could challenge and subvert the "modern social imaginary." This is because we have contended that this social imaginary lies behind the phenomenon of "burdened agency" we increasingly face today. Hauerwas has focused our attention on the relationship between the practices and formation of community and the grammar and language that precedes the concrete ethical dilemmas we encounter. In this final section, we turn to a community whose way of life and grammar have deeply influenced Hauerwas and that illustrates what it means to live an "ethic of dispossession."

It is hard to overstate the impression the L'Arche community had on Hauerwas.[75] For all his attention to the Church/world distinction and his robust ecclesiology, a common retort to Hauerwas is the following: "Show me this church of which you speak." Perhaps more than anywhere else, Hauerwas can (and does) point to L'Arche communities as "an example of what it means to be church."[76] For they represent for Hauerwas the type of community required to sustain the practices and skills needed for "living gently in a violent world,"[77] virtues like patience, which is essential for living with those who are not mentally or physically agile.

Of particular importance in his appreciation for L'Arche is the way in which the communities cultivate an awareness of vulnerability and dependence, not just for those within the community labeled "disabled" but for all. Although most of us do not have significant intellectual disabilities, we all experience infancy—and many will experience old age—along with the sense of vulnerability that accompanies it. These stages are the two "golden ages of our lives," for the "vulnerability we experience by being young or old creates the condition that makes the work of the Holy Spirit possible. To be young or old is to lack the means—as the disabled do—to disguise our desire to be loved. Yet that 'weakness' enables the Holy Spirit to act toward the young, old and the disabled in a special way."[78] L'Arche communities are communities of the joyfully dispossessed because their members cannot deny their neediness. Although L'Arche typically eschews the language of the medical lexicon, those who dwell within these communities are "patients" in the truest sense—for they are those who know and recognize themselves as *sufferers* of the limits of bodily creaturehood.

It would be difficult to overstate the significance of the virtue of patience for Hauerwas. Although Hauerwas repeatedly notes the interconnection of the virtues, he returns to patience again and again. Patience, it turns out, has direct implications, for Hauerwas, for the way Christians approach the use of health care at the end of life. For example, Hauerwas finds it morally significant that although medicine has become increasingly defined in terms of professionalism (e.g., the "professional-client relationship"), we have nevertheless generally retained the use of the term "patient."

According to Hauerwas (and Charles Pinches), "the retention of 'patients' in medicine and the continued practice of patience by patients is key to the good practice of medicine."[79] Moreover, "Christians are called to be a patient people, in health and in sickness. . . . If Christians are faithful, they will be . . . the most patient of patients" (349). Hence, the reason why Hauerwas finds L'Arche to be a picture of the church. Dispossessed of their need for control, Christians have time to let the other be other. According to the authors, "if Christians have anything to offer, it is to be the patients who embody the virtue of Christian patience" (349). But Christians will not be patient in illness or at their dying if they have not first learned to be patient in health. Fortunately, "God has given us resources for recovering the practice of patience" (364). Among these are our bodies, complete with their finitude and fragility, their unwillingness and inability to simply bend themselves to our will in any and every situation. Second, we are given the gift of relationships and community. The "unavoidability of the other" provides not only an external limitation to my will, but an occasion to love the other as the one who fittingly confronts me with their own being.[80] Finally, we are given the gift of "time and space for the acquisition of habits that come from worthy activities." Such activities require time and attention, especially insofar as we learn to pass them on to our children by patiently providing the opportunity for them to learn from us. The Christian practice of patience also opens up into witness, for "if Christians could be such patient patients . . . we might well stand as witnesses to our non-Christian neighbor of the truth of the story of God's patient care of God's creatures" (355–56).

As Christians learn the virtue of patience through the practice of dispossession, they become better prepared for the challenges that they are likely to confront in navigating the use of medicine at the end of life. In particular, they become the sorts of persons for whom the following collect from the *Book of Common Prayer* will become comprehensible: "This is another day, O Lord. I know not what it will bring forth, but make me ready, Lord, for whatever it may be. If I am to stand up, help me to stand bravely. If I am to sit still, help me to sit quietly. If I am to lie low, help me do it patiently. If I am to do nothing, let me do it gallantly. Make these words more than words, and give me the Spirit of Jesus, Amen." "Doing nothing gallantly" only makes sense as an option when patients reject the desperate attempt to defeat death.[81] Christians should be able to see "that accepting the fatedness of our ending is a way of affirming the trustworthiness of God's care for us." As a result, the Christian "will not fight [her] death nor the death of others when it cannot be avoided." What is needed, and what Christians should have, is "a language of finitude, a way of talking decently about the limits of human life, a way of saying why and under what circumstances death is natural. . . . It may be that we must be willing to die a good deal earlier"[82] than others.

As Iris Murdoch insightfully noted, "at crucial moments of choice most of the business of choosing is already over."[83] The moral life includes far more than the decisions that we make—for Murdoch, what happens between dilemmas and decisions is far more important for the character of our action in the world. This is the point that has been driven home in the current chapter. Hauerwas draws together connections between notions of moral agency, virtue and formation, and narrative and communal practices.

One question, however, remains—namely, what are the prospects for virtuous formation that Hauerwas describes if the analysis offered in chapter 1 is accurate? For if we experience our agency in dying in a particularly reflexive and individualistic way, it is at least partly because we struggle to make sense of our living and dying according to the norms and stories of stabilizing (what Zygmunt Bauman called "solid") institutions. And the reasons for such deinsitutionalization of dying are deeply entrenched. What is needed are ad hoc persistent acts of renarration that remind people of the moral grammar that is already embedded within their communal practices to challenge the dominant social imaginary. In the next chapter, I will turn to ecclesial practices in the Christian tradition, articulating their relation to notions of agency in dying that have been developed throughout this book. In doing so, I will note where such practices seem to offer resources for challenging the status quo.

SIX

Prayer, Baptism, and Eucharist

MORTALITY, MORAL AGENCY, AND CHRISTIAN PRACTICES

The central narrative of the Christian faith revolves around a first-century Galilean peasant who, according to the Apostles' Creed, "suffered under [Roman governor] Pontius Pilate, was crucified, died, and was buried . . . [and] descended to the dead." It should be no surprise, then, that the central images and practices of the Christian faith also revolve around death—specifically, the singular death of this one who "died for us" (Rom 5:8; 1 Thess 5:10; compare Rom 8:34; Gal 3:13; Eph 5:2; Titus 2:14; 1 John 3:16). Yet Christians do not often recognize and appreciate this truth.

Of course, Jesus's death may only be understood in light of his later resurrection; Christians do not celebrate Christ's death as such. As Paul makes clear, the fact of the resurrection makes all the difference: "If Christ has not been raised, your faith is futile and you are still in your sins. Then those who have fallen asleep in Christ have perished. If in Christ we have hope in this life only, we are of all people most to be pitied" (1 Cor 15:17–19). But for all its importance, the resurrection does not eliminate but rather illuminates the centrality of Jesus's saving death.[1] As the Apostle Thomas discovered in the upper room (John 20:24–28), the Risen Christ bears the marks of crucifixion in his resurrected body. The Risen Jesus is eternally the Crucified One. And this is necessarily so, for nothing that has not died can be resurrected.[2]

This chapter spells out and makes explicit theological understandings of death that are embedded in the practices of prayer, baptism, and Eucharist. Because human beings are not, at the most basic level, "brains on sticks" but rather "bundles of loves," the forms of agency described so far (spirituality of martyrdom, creaturely finitude, and an ethic of dispossession) are more caught than taught. Indeed, they must be cultivated and inculcated over time through habit-forming practices. Therefore, these practices provide resources for generating new ways of understanding agency in dying and human agency as such. Turning to the practices of the church, it will be important to give Jesus's death its due. In a society that consistently denies the reality of death in which the dying are typically sequestered from the larger community, the fact that the Christian church so consistently brings to mind through its practices the death of Jesus is significant.

In turning to practices, I want to avoid certain misconceptions. The practices mentioned—though not all technically "sacraments"—each have a sacramental quality to them. They are each outward signs of an inward grace, which affect what they signify. I want to be careful, however, to avoid the illusion that these religious practices can be understood primarily as strategies of self-improvement or Foucauldian technologies of the self. Especially in this context where the emphasis is on how these particular practices can challenge our very notions of self-control and self-possession, such a misunderstanding would be unfortunate.

It is also important not to focus exclusively on practices that occur near or at the moment of death (as happens, for example, in certain empirical studies of the effectiveness of prayer or anointing). As M. Therese Lysaught points out, "the power and importance of sacramental practices lie . . . not solely or primarily in their utilization in the immediate context of end-of-life care . . . [but rather] in the ongoing, lifelong immersion of Christians in these practices in the context of the church. Sacramental practices serve to form congregations and worshipers—in an ongoing, continuous, recursive way—to be the body of Christ in the world in their living, their working, and their dying."[3] Without caution, sacramental practices can become subsumed within the modern social imaginary rather than the other way around. Sacraments have an effect in the world, but they are not "health technologies."[4] Rather, the effect that one may hope to see is a more gradual, lifelong transformation on the level of comportment or posture. In Lysaught's words, "As we meet this love in the Eucharist and the sacraments, we are—by grace—transformed (act by act by act) into the image of Christ so that we, too, can incarnate that kenotic love in the world. God's love is to become the shape of our lives."[5] The following kenotic practices may shape one's posture toward suffering, illness, and death. If one cannot ultimately unburden her agency, she may at least bear it well.

PRAYER: EMPOWERING DEPENDENCE

Prayer is counterintuitive. In it, transcendence and fullness are found through the emptying of the self. Mary prays, "Here I am, the servant of the LORD. Let it be with me according to your word." Jesus prays, "Nevertheless, not my will but yours be done." The Church prays "Our Father in heaven, hallowed be *your* name. *Your* kingdom come, *your* will be done . . . for *yours* are the kingdom, power, and glory forever, amen." As theologian Sarah Coakley notes, prayers like these involve "*displacing one's self* or waiting for something else to arrive."[6] Or as Merold Westphal puts it, prayer is "the deepest decentering of the self, deep enough to begin dismantling or, if you like, deconstructing that burning preoccupation with myself."[7]

Prayer is a practice that shapes both an individual's self-identity and her posture toward the world, what David Kelsey calls one's "existential how."[8] This process of formation is perhaps best exemplified in the fourteenth-century handbook *The Cloud of Unknowing*. This work was written by an anonymous monk to direct a young novice in the "work of contemplation."[9] The author offers a series of directives for a spiritual practice of apophatic prayer, or prayer by way of negation (*via negativa*). The main insight of this work can be summed up in the words of Saint Denis, quoted by the author: "The truly divine knowledge of God is that which is known by unknowing." Because of the ontological and epistemological gulf between God and humanity, the one who thinks she can reach God through "intellectual labor" is "perilously deluded" (16–17). There will always be a dark "cloud of unknowing" preventing one from "seeing [God] clearly by the light of understanding in reason." Fortunately, though incomprehensible to the intellect, God is "entirely comprehensible" to the "loving power" within each and every person (13). "It is love alone that can reach God in this life, and not knowing" (27).

The goal of prayer, then, is the cultivation of one's desire for God and the orientation of one's will toward God. To pray rightly, the novice should "lift up [her] heart to God with a humble impulse of love, and have [God alone] as [her] aim" (10). She should be careful not to fix her attention on any created thing—not even herself or the blessings that God bestows on her. She should even avoid thinking about God's character or perfections, which can only imperfectly describe God by way of analogy with created things. She should press down all thoughts of created things beneath a "cloud of forgetting," should "step above [each one] stalwartly but lovingly, and with a devout, pleasing, impulsive love strive to pierce that darkness above [her], to smite upon that thick cloud of unknowing with a sharp dart of longing love" (20). If a thought should arise, of any sort, she should say in her heart "You have no part to play. . . . Go down again" into the cloud of forgetting. This exercise requires no words, but allowing for the difficulty of wordless thought, the author makes a concession: "If you like, you can have this reaching out [to God] wrapped up and enfolded in a single word. So as to have a better grasp of it, take just a little word, of one syllable rather than two, for the shorter it is, the better it is in agreement with this exercise of the spirit. Such a one is the word 'God' or the word 'love.' . . . With this word you are to beat upon this cloud and this darkness above you. With this word you are to strike down every kind of thought under the cloud of forgetting" (22–23).

In her book *Powers and Submissions*,[10] Coakley helpfully unpacks the dynamics of moral agency and identity formation that are embedded within apophatic prayer practices like the one just described. She notes how nondiscursive and nonconceptual prayer (what she calls "silent prayer") involve a renunciation of the notion of control, a patient waiting, and a decentering of the self and its desires in hopes (and expectation) of grace drawing the prayer toward mystical union with the divine.

There are many forms of prayer in the Christian tradition that fit this description, not all of them strictly wordless. One may think, for example, of the Quaker prayer meeting, the practice of "centering prayer," the charismatic experience of glossolalia, or the Eastern Orthodox Jesus Prayer (repeatedly, "Lord Jesus Christ, Son of God, have mercy on me, a sinner"). As with *The Cloud of Unknowing*, each of these practices enacts a form of thought that is nondiscursive and therefore in some sense passive. For example, as Coakley explains, in reciting the Jesus Prayer, the aim is not necessarily to focus on the meaning of each word but rather to "use repetitive but mechanical 'acts'. . . . not as the prayer, but as a sort of accompanying 'drone' to keep the imagination occupied. . . . Not only is the imagination thus mechanically stilled, but the 'drone' also helps prevent the mind from operating discursively; thus the (empty) intellect is left facing a 'blank,' with the will gently holding it there."[11] According to Coakley, these practices enact a "spiritual extension of Christic *kenosis*" (emptying) because the one who thus prays must refuse from the outset a grasping, controlling mentality. This "involves an ascetical commitment of some subtlety, a regular and willed *practice* of ceding and responding to the divine."[12] Coakley calls this "gentle space-making."

The adjective "gentle" is key, for Coakley's treatment of silent prayer in *Powers and Submissions* comprises an extended refutation of the critiques of feminist theologians like Daphne Hampson, who suggests that "for women, the theme of self-emptying and self-abnegation is far from helpful as a [spiritual] paradigm."[13] It is one thing for someone who enjoys social prestige and privilege, including some measure of economic and political stability, to be told that he should embrace contingency and vulnerability as an expression of faith in Christ's ultimate victory and trustworthiness. It is another thing altogether to tell this to someone who has very little power from which she may be "dispossessed" and who already experiences the threat of "vulnerability" in spades.[14] Therefore, it is significant that the encounter that takes place in silent prayer is "not an invitation to be battered; nor is its silence a silenc*ing*. . . . God . . . neither shouts nor forces, let alone 'obliterates.'" This form of "self-emptying" is not simply an abnegation of the self but rather "the place of the self's transformation and expansion into God."[15]

While acknowledging the power of the critique from the standpoint of feminism, I would affirm Sarah Coakley's suggestion that the Christian doctrine of kenosis may nevertheless be affirmed and embraced from the perspective of feminism, so long as the doctrine is properly construed. Indeed, as Coakley argues, "some version[s] of *kenosis* [are] not only compatible with feminism, but vital to a distinctly Christian manifestation of it, a manifestation which does not eschew, but embraces, the spiritual paradoxes of 'losing one's life in order to save it.'"[16] For, properly understood, the openness and vulnerability that is central to this kenotic theology is that which is open and vulnerable to the Divine. This special form of human vulnerability is normative precisely because it carves out a space for God's empowering of the human being.

Graham Ward has developed a similar account of kenosis from Gregory of Nyssa's notion of suffering as the "wounding of love."[17] Ward argues that a theological emphasis on kenosis (emptying) must be balanced in equal measure by the Pauline concept of *plerosis* (filling up). Ward exposits Paul's use of *pleroo* as a "theological reflection of the economics of divine power with respect to embodiment in Christ . . . a reflection upon divinity as it manifests itself in the concrete historicity of the death, burial, and resurrection of Jesus the Christ."[18] There exists an intra-divine "passion," a love relationship of unity in difference and difference in unity, between Father, Son, and Holy Spirit that involves a continual dynamic of kenosis and *plerosis*. It is an "economy of that loving which incarnates the very logic of sacrifice as the endless giving (which is also a giving-up, a *kenosis*) and the endless reception (which is also an opening up towards the other in order to be filled)."[19] Ward here unites traditional notions of agape and eros as two elements of one love relationship—without thereby gendering these notions as masculine and feminine. The human is most fully human in a kenotic posture (which mimics God's own) that simultaneously opens itself up to fulfillment and plenitude. It is precisely in the self's kenotic and patient silence that it acknowledges its creaturely dependence on the divine. In the practice of silent prayer, the one who prays relates to God as she was created to relate to God, with an awareness and acknowledgment of dependence on God for every breath.

To illustrate how prayer reshapes moral agency in a way that subverts the modern social imaginary, consider the Physician's Vocation Program, an elective track for medical students launched in 2012 at the Loyola University Chicago Stritch School of Medicine.[20] Students who opt into this program "explore the intersection of their faith and their professional development as physicians through a program of coursework, prayer, and reflection."[21] Wasson et al. describe the program this way: "The Physician's Vocation Program seeks to form physicians who will bring to the practice of medicine not only technical proficiencies and business efficiencies, but also human wisdom and compassion. . . . [The] program does so through the use of a habit of reflection rooted in a spiritual tradition some five hundred years old—but ever new to those who employ it."[22]

The spiritual tradition in this case is the practice of Ignatian spirituality, the foundation of the Jesuit Catholic tradition. Ignatian spirituality is based on the writings of Ignatius of Loyola, whose "foundational spiritual insight was that God was present to him through the routine elements of his daily life. This observation led him to understand God to be found 'in all things.' What is needed for a healthy spiritual life, then, is a habit of reflection that attends to God's presence or absence in the events of a day. The root of Ignatian reflection is first a process of personal introspection that moves to a decision about how one ought to love and to serve God in all things."[23]

This prayer practice (called the examen) is paired with coursework that emphasizes "the spiritual roots of medicine's practice: the experience of illness, the possibility of healing and hope, what it means to be embodied and destined to die, and how one reconciles the claim of a loving God with a world that suffers."[24] The examen involves a combination of attention, memory, and silent waiting. Likewise, it teaches that the greatest form of empowerment occurs when one is in a posture of openness and vulnerability to the divine. The examen, then, constitutes a kenotic activity of gentle space-making that enacts the truest form of humanity before God. It is a form of what Iris Murdoch would call "unselfing," which prefigures and anticipates the great unselfing that occurs for each person when they die. It is a practice of *dis*possession.

BAPTISM: THE FIRST ACT OF CHRISTIAN MARTYRDOM

Baptism is one of the central rites of the Christian church. The symbolism associated with baptism is complex and multilayered—with differing emphases across various denominations and traditions. For some, baptism primarily represents initiation into the people of God, the church, in much the same way that circumcision did among the Hebrew people (compare Col 2:11–12). Others emphasize cleansing and renewal through the washing away of sin (compare Acts 22:16). Still others see in baptism a clear expression of the unity of the church hidden in Christ (compare Eph 4:5; 1 Cor 12:13).

Despite this multiplicity of meanings, the central, controlling metaphor of baptism is the believer's "dying and rising" in Christ. "Do you not know that all of us who have been baptized into Christ Jesus were baptized into his death? We were buried therefore with him by baptism into death, in order that, just as Christ was raised from the dead by the glory of the Father, we too might walk in newness of life. For if we have been united with him in a death like his, we shall be united with him in a resurrection like his" (Rom 6:3–5). Baptism is a putting to death, a burial (Col 2:12) of the sinner—only on the far side of which is new life found. Jesus himself spoke of his own coming death as his "baptism" in which his disciples would share through their own suffering and death (e.g., Matt 20:22–23; Mark 10:38–39; Luke 12:50). In the characteristically bracing words of Martin Luther, "Your baptism is nothing less than grace clutching you by the throat: a grace-full throttling, by which your sin is submerged in order that ye may remain under grace. Come thus to thy baptism. Give thyself up to be drowned in baptism and killed by the mercy of thy dear God, saying: 'Drown me and throttle me, dear Lord, for henceforth I will gladly die to sin with thy dear son.'"[25]

Submerged beneath the waters, we die; lifted out of the water, we arise to new life. We rise also to a completely new identity. The identity change that is signified by baptism is drastic and total—it is no less than a death and rebirth, a new creation (2 Cor 5:17). The baptismal identity is fundamentally defined by one's relation to Jesus Christ rather than the self. The baptized Christian is baptized into Christ's death, to arise in Christ's resurrection—in short, her new identity is thoroughly in Christ. Therefore, Rowan Williams describes the church as the "community of those who have been 'immersed' in Jesus' life, overwhelmed by it. . . . [The baptized] have disappeared under the surface of Christ's love and reappeared as different people. The waters close over their heads, and then, like the old world rising out of watery chaos in the first chapter of the Bible, out comes a new world. So when the Church baptizes people, it says what it is and what sort of life its people live."[26]

Elsewhere, Williams draws together the connection between baptism, death, and identity by arguing that baptism confers a "martyrial identity" on the Christian.[27] Incorporation into Christ's body (i.e., his death and resurrection) is not simply a personal or ecclesial act but also a political act. The baptismal identity is one that witnesses to the lordship of Christ rather than the lordship of the empire. In the context of the ancient church, such a declaration of loyalty could get you killed. Baptism, as placing one's life and future in the hands of the crucified and risen lamb, is an act that finds its final expression in what we now call martyrdom. It is "for the specific commission to die at the hands of the powerful of this earth, to realize God's power through the gift of one's own life to him . . . so that the washing of the convert becomes an identification with [Jesus's] death, [his] gift and [his] empowering" to be faithful unto death.[28] As Lysaught notes, "baptism prefigures . . . martyrdom" just as martyrdom, the "second baptism," perfects and completes the baptismal identity.[29]

What does such an existence look like in the mundane realities of the everyday? There is no way to comprehensively determine the answer to that question in an a priori fashion. It must be discerned by the individual Christian as she navigates the particular circumstances of her situation and context. But obvious tensions exist between the martyr's view of agency and the understanding of agency in the modern social imaginary. The latter is predicated on an association between human dignity and the efficacious control of nature and the material world, which allows for the minimization of the effects of natural contingency and the possibility of suffering. "The martyr's agency," according to Brad Gregory, "depended on relinquishing control, their strength upon a naked admission of their utter impotence and total dependence upon God."[30] It is quite possible that faithfulness could require choices of Christians that seem at odds with prevailing "wisdom" and ideological assumptions. For example, it may be the case that Christians choose to continue upholding the moral importance of the distinction between killing and letting die (even though such a distinction has been challenged philosophically and is difficult to apply in particular contexts), if only to preserve the sense that instrumental and efficient control need not extend over any and every aspect of our living and dying.

Another point of tension arises with respect to the concept of "identity." Within the expressivist strand of the modern social imaginary at least, authenticity is a central value. Baptism, however, expresses the fact that theologically understood, the Christian identity is "eccentric"—derived from without rather than within.[31] Christ's life, death, and resurrection is mysteriously more fundamental to my identity—if indeed I am in Christ—than my own deepest sense of self. This is not to say that Christianity is against authenticity. But it may challenge the notion that appeals to authenticity in arguments about physician-assisted suicide or in hospice practices should constitute "hypergoods," which trump, for example, more communitarian concerns. For example, Michael Banner argues that the common rhetorical trope of "death before death," most commonly applied to persons with advanced Alzheimer's disease, "risks perpetuating a culturally influential, yet very limited notion of what constitutes the presence or continuation of selfhood."[32] It is sometimes said of such persons, "He is a shell of his former self" or "It's as if mother is no longer there." But Banner draws on anthropologist Janelle Taylor to make the point that care for Alzheimer's patients is in fact marked by the practice of continued recognition—even, perhaps especially, in cases when the patient has lost the ability to recognize others.[33] Sometimes with great personal difficulty, family members continue to spend time with the person with Alzheimer's, treating them according to the values and preferences they have previously held. They make sure that Grandma has her favorite perfume each day or that Grandpa is able to shave himself or wear his favorite lapel pin.[34] They continue to use personal names, honorifics, or nicknames as they address loved ones. In everyday practices of care, they are able to uphold the patient in her identity in a way that is analogous with God's upholding of our own identity.

A final tension worth noting regards differing evaluations of natural limits. Mark Medley describes how Williams applies the logic of baptismal identity in the quotidian realities of daily life by shifting the emphasis from a heroic act to a "nondramatic" spiritual discipline: "While literal martyrdom is a political and spiritual act which fulfills the baptismal confession, martyrdom can also be understood as a spiritual discipline, a form of *askesis* that calls Christians to adjust one's bodily existence in the world so as to perform the radically new way of life that God has wrought in Christ's *kenosis*."[35] In other words, the baptismal identity results in what Nathan Kerr has called a "sociality of dispossession."[36]

If this is correct, renewed attention to the symbolic logic of baptism could generate new ways of imagining the process of dispossession called "aging" or "old age." Returning to Banner, "the problem with our long dying in general is just, of course, that it seems like death in slow motion: we are totally undone by death, but in our long dying, we are undone bit by bit."[37] The long dwindling that increasingly characterizes death is a process of moving toward dependencies and away from capabilities. It is a process of surrender. But the "surrender of the self" is nothing new to a baptismal people. They have already surrendered to "death before death," both in the event of baptism itself and in the living out of their baptismal and martyrial identity. Gracefully accepting the dispossession of old age because one has already been dispossessed of self in baptism is a form of martyrdom for the church today. For the church to embrace this transformative practice would challenge dominant cultural assumptions about aging and disability. But it would require the courage of our older persons to age publicly so that their example of graceful dispossession can truly stand as a witness for the edification of the Church.

For the Christian who has already suffered the most relevant death in being buried with Jesus through baptism, the rest of life takes on the character of superabundance and gift. In all of these ways, every baptized Christian brings her baptismal identity to bear on her professional roles and responsibilities as well as her familial, social, and personal relationships. Although baptism signifies an identity change that is so total as to constitute a death and rebirth, we should not therefore conclude that it erases all other concerns and projects we might find ourselves implicated in. The transcendent and eccentric identity conferred through baptism, however, critically shapes and constrains the prevailing identity markers of the modern social imaginary.

This brings up an important question: If baptism is a singular action, not to be repeated, is it possible for it to truly do the work of altering our self-understanding in such a profound manner? This question is especially acute for traditions that affirm infant baptism, for how, exactly, is baptism supposed to challenge dominant social imaginaries if one cannot even remember it happening?

A theological response might begin by alluding to the work of the Holy Spirit, which cannot be anticipated or controlled but which is associated with baptism throughout the New Testament. Baptism is not a "technology of the self" so much as a "means of grace." Nevertheless, the church has long emphasized the remembrance of baptism as a communal practice.

This does not refer to a remembrance of the actual event but rather the remembrance of the fact that one has been baptized, calling to mind all that is entailed by it. In some denominations, such remembrance is aided by the lighting of a baptismal candle each year on the anniversary of one's baptism. Another aid to such remembrance is the regular public performance of baptism, especially when such a performance becomes an occasion for repeating and affirming baptismal vows. We might ask what it would mean for the performance of baptism and reaffirmation of vows to be truly public? And a related question we might pose is, what would happen if we tried to bring the practice of baptism into the clinic? One problem with such an idea is that it would most likely be messy and quite disruptive. Perhaps, however, it is in the very disruption of medical and technological efficiency that the practice of baptism speaks its prophetic word.

EUCHARIST: BECOMING THE BROKEN BODY OF CHRIST

If baptism signifies the Christian's union with Christ's death and resurrection, in the Eucharist she is drawn further into this mysterious reality. "Take and eat, this is my body. . . . Drink of it, all of you. This is my blood of the covenant, which is poured out for many for the forgiveness of sins" (Matt 26:26–28; compare Luke 22:19–20). As with baptism, the symbolism here is rich and multifaceted. The Eucharist has been understood variously as a memorial, as a proclamation, as a meal, and as an eschatological foretaste. Each of these is true. The Eucharist, or Lord's Supper, is a memorial by which the church recalls Christ's sacrifice on the cross. It is a way of calling to mind the fact that "nothing but the blood of Jesus" can ultimately save. When one is tempted in a million different ways to make oneself into one's own savior, the regular practice of the Eucharist is a desperately needed reminder that one is saved by grace.

But the Eucharist is more than an aid to individual Christians' recollection. It is also a public performance, an act of proclamation (*kerygma*). "Whenever you eat this bread and drink this cup *you proclaim* the Lord's death until he comes" (1 Cor 11:28). This makes the Eucharist a martyrial act in much the same way that baptism is. It is an act of witness unto death.

William Cavanaugh argues that historically, "the eucharist [had been] inextricably linked with martyrdom in the life of the church," especially as each powerfully enacts a self-giving ethic that reveals, and thereby subverts, the violence hidden deep in the heart of the empire.

> In the Christian tradition, both the martyrs and the eucharist participate, through the power of the Holy Spirit, in the sacrifice of Christ in such a way that a body of people is built up and made visible. In this body of people, the body of Christ, the powers of darkness are resisted because the truth about their violence is revealed in the violence they inflict on the body. Martyrdom and the eucharist reveal the irruption of Christ's kingdom into history, a revelation that both judges the divisions that exist and, at the same time, points hopefully forward to the day when such divisions will be overcome.[38]

Beyond remembering and proclaiming the Lord's death, however, the Eucharist does something more: it makes Christ's death and resurrection present in us. It is the meal, which by incorporating us into Jesus's broken body, gives us life. Jesus is the bread of life "who comes down from heaven and gives life to the world" (John 6:33). In John's gospel, Jesus assures his followers, "Unless you eat the flesh of the Son of Man and drink his blood, you have no life in you. Whoever eats my flesh and drinks my blood has eternal life, and I will raise them up at the last day. For my flesh is real food and my blood is real drink. Whoever eats my flesh and drinks my blood remains in me, and I in them" (John 6:53–58). As Augustine noted, however, Jesus's flesh is a very peculiar sort of food. By eating, we do not metabolize the bread and wine into us so much as we are metabolized into them.[39] As the church celebrates the Eucharist, it is literally *in*corporated into the body of Christ—but importantly, into the body that is "broken" and "poured out." The people of God are reminded in the Eucharist that they are marked by (Christ's own) sacrifice and kenotic, self-emptying love rather than the hubris of spiritual triumphalism.

Finally, the Eucharist points not only backward to Christ's sacrifice but also forward to the eschatological wedding feast in the new creation. In the Eucharist, we "proclaim the Lord's death until he comes," which is to say that we do so in hopeful anticipation of his final presence and ultimate redemption. The Eucharist is a foretaste of the kingdom of heaven. It is also an anticipation of the perfection of humanity. In it, the believer receives Jesus Christ, the perfect human, himself. And in receiving Christ, she is mysteriously drawn into the fullness of his glorious image. There is cause for celebration and rejoicing at the Eucharist. It would be wrong, however, to imagine this perfection simply as a reversal of human death and suffering—a triumphant "never mind to all that." For as the Risen Christ bears the marks of crucifixion, the triumphant One seated on the throne (Rev 7:17) is also the lamb "who was slain from the foundation of the world" (Rev 13:8).

The last section considered baptism as a quotidian practice. Similarly, Ellen Concannon proposes that we might begin to develop a eucharistic identity in everyday life by recognizing how the Eucharist exemplifies and establishes the perfection of human freedom. Drawing on Rahner's notion of a "fundamental option," she suggests that true freedom is demonstrated in one's openness to God and in one's willingness to live by and for God. It is in saying yes to the prior Yes of God that one's freedom is made complete. The deepest and truest yes to God ever seen occurred in Christ's self-giving sacrifice on the cross and in Jesus's Gethsemane prayer, "Nevertheless, not my will but Thy will be done" (Luke 22:42). This perfected human freedom is both manifested and promised in the Eucharist. In the broken bread and poured-out wine, we look back to Jesus's example and forward to our own destiny. Or more precisely, in the Eucharist Jesus's sacrifice is brought forward in time and our destiny is brought backward in time, as each meets us in the present moment. For this reason, Concannon states, "Definitive human freedom is eschatological and thus also Eucharistic."[40]

Accordingly, this view of freedom attributes a special importance to suffering and death. It is at death that one's fundamental orientation toward God is finally and definitively demonstrated, but this orientation is prefigured in how one responds to all the "little deaths" brought about by more mundane experiences of suffering. "I die every day" (1 Cor 15:31), exclaimed the Apostle Paul. The Christian is buried with Christ in baptism and transformed into the broken body of Christ through the Eucharist. Especially in Paul's letters we see that those who identify with Christ's suffering and death in this way may experience their own suffering as a mystical participation in Christ's own suffering. "I carry the marks of Jesus branded on my body" (Gal 6:17). "We suffer with him so that we may also be glorified with him" (Rom 8:17; compare 2 Cor 1:5–11). "I want to know

Christ ... and the sharing of his sufferings by becoming like him in his death" (Phil 3:10; compare 2 Cor 13:4; Gal 2:19). "We are afflicted in every way, but not crushed ... , always carrying in the body the death of Jesus, so that the life of Jesus may also be made visible in our bodies. For while we live, we are always being given up to death for Jesus' sake, so that the life of Jesus may be made visible in our mortal flesh" (2 Cor 4:8–11).

The Christian approaches the altar with empty hands, turned up in a posture of receptive and open submission to what God has for him, which is ultimately Godself. What he receives is a sign of the death before which he must ultimately submit and which he anticipates in the *prolixitas mortis* (Gregory the Great) that occurs throughout his entire life. Every Eucharist is an invitation to follow Jesus in his submission unto death: but this very same invitation is extended in every moment of life and perhaps most acutely in every experience of suffering. Therefore, the Eucharist is best understood "not [as] something other than the everyday, but rather [as] most especially the everyday in all its mundaneness."[41]

The frequent practice of the Eucharist holds immense promise for shaping a cultural imaginary that resists the dominant logics of medicalized dying and for the generation of new visions for common end-of-life practices. A people shaped by the Eucharist cannot long deny their mortality and vulnerability.[42] In the "visible words" of bread and wine, we are confronted with the fact that Jesus did not shun mortality but subjected himself to it to become what we are so that we might be made like him.

Our limitations present no impediment to the love of God that transcends even death. God's love meets us and nourishes us precisely in and through the brokenness of his human flesh, made present to us in the Eucharist. A eucharistic imagination is characterized by union in brokenness, which allows for a reevaluation of bodily limitations and even of various forms of disability, dependency, and decline. The "body" shaped by the practices of Eucharist, insofar as it is being drawn into union with Christ, is always already a broken body. In the words of Lysaught, "As we enter ever more deeply and increasingly into the worship of the Triune God, we risk becoming ever more transformed into the image of the crucified Christ."[43] This is true whether we imagine such a "body" as an individual person's physical frame or whether we are considering the corporate body of believers, the "body of Christ" (1 Cor 12:27; compare Rom 12:5; Eph 3:6, 5:23; Col 1:18, 24).

In recent years, valuable insights from disability studies have been increasingly appreciated by theologians and Christian ethicists. One important insight for theological anthropology is the fact that none of us "is ever more than temporarily able-bodied."[44] The line distinguishing persons with disabilities from those who are "normally abled" is permeable, and most of us, whether through illness or old age, will share the experience of struggling with physical and mental limitations. Acknowledging this fact moves the experience of limitation into the center of our reflection on what it means to live as embodied human creatures. As Deborah Creamer notes, "Disability is not something that exists solely as a negative experience of limitation but [is] rather . . . an intrinsic, unsurprising, and valuable element of human limited-ness."[45] Although we tend to "deny the normality of limits in all of our lives . . . limits are a normal and unsurprising aspect of life."[46] In other words, recalling Karl Barth, "the finitude of our being belongs to our God-given nature" (III.2, 627).

This leads to another key insight of disability studies: in light of the centrality of human limitedness, preconceived notions about normalcy and flourishing may need to be revised. Limits do not necessarily inhibit flourishing but rather provide the context in which flourishing, theologically understood, does or does not occur. A eucharistic imagination holds an expanded, and at times counterintuitive, picture of well-being and so will not simply accept the models supplied by the dominant social imaginary. Flourishing, or well-being, is not to be equated with "biostatistical normalcy," "species-typical functioning," or "capabilities." To be nourished by the Eucharist is to become, by grace through faith, the broken body of Jesus Christ. This is not to say that Christians seek brokenness for the sake of brokenness, suffering for the sake of suffering. They do not. But the presence or absence of suffering and brokenness, in body or spirit, presents no obstacle to our being "conformed to the image" of Jesus Christ (Rom 8:29; compare Eph 4:15; 2 Cor 3:18), who bears his bodily brokenness into his risen and glorious existence (John 20:27) and who imparts his broken-yet-risen identity to his church in the bread and wine at Communion.

In this light, it is instructive to consider the roots of hospice and palliative care. That Dame Cicely Saunders introduced a revolutionary new form of medicine when she began St. Christopher's Hospice in 1967 is generally recognized. But the fact that she did so as a self-conscious expression of her

Christian faith and vocation is less appreciated. In fact, Darren Henson has argued that it was "the very practice of the Christian life in [the] liturgical and sacramental life of the Church [that] gave rise to Saunders' vision of palliative care."[47] In the context of regular Bible study and Christian communal living, a young Cicely Saunders initially discerned the call to care for the needs of the dying in their "total pain," which includes much more than physical pain. As Saunders matured in her Christian faith and attended medical school, she continued to work with patients at a home for the dying, St. Joseph's Hospice in Hackney, run by the Irish Sisters of Charity, a Roman Catholic religious order. These experiences and others were formative for her own vision of a new model of end-of-life care. This vision called for a new, hybrid institution, simultaneously "medical" and "religious." Although in her public speaking engagements she tended to downplay the religious foundations of St. Christopher's Hospice, the centrality of Christian convictions is evidenced in the founding documents as well as in the very architectural choices that were made upon its creation. According to Lysaught, Saunders "sought to design St. Christopher's Hospice with the chapel in the center of the building so that visually, structurally, and infrastructurally, the Eucharist would be at the center of their lives and work together and 'Christ's victory over pain and death' could 'radiate out from the Chapel into every part of the corporate life.'"[48] Indeed, in a letter composed shortly after the opening of St. Christopher's, Saunders writes, "Today we are having our first Communion service, with two patients down from the ward in their beds, so we have really gone straight on with the important things."[49] As the quotation indicates, the regular practice of the Eucharist and other Christian practices served as a reminder of Christ's "victory over pain and death." Henson notes how the practice of the Eucharist shaped what would become palliative care medicine:

> The daily rhythm of liturgical prayer makes the religious mindful of the rising of the sun and its setting, the creation of the world and its final fulfillment at the end of time, the birth and life of Jesus as well as his passion, death and resurrection. This ongoing reminder and celebration of God's omnipresence and fidelity provides the religious with a particular understanding of life and death. In turn, it influences and animates the care offered to those enduring the vulnerabilities of illness and the

burdens of dying. Because they had been formed with the Catholic imagination to be attuned to the presence of Christ in the eucharistic liturgy, it was a natural step for superiors to urge their sister and brother caregivers to see the mystical body of Christ in the patients for whom they cared.[50]

CONCLUSION: THE PROMISE OF CHRISTIAN PRACTICES

The practices covered in this chapter—prayer, baptism, and Eucharist—center on notions of agency that are more native to Christian soil (e.g., martyrdom, kenosis, dispossession, receptivity, and submission) than to the modern social imaginary. Given the right narrative and the proper concepts and grammar of agency and trained into that narrative through practices, patients (who engage with hospice and palliative care) and physicians (who give such care) will have a renewed understanding of what is occurring, one that does not perpetuate unhelpful assumptions about moral agency that underlie the dynamics that lead to burdened agency.

Christians who are embedded in health-care practices, either as caregivers or patients, will find themselves enmeshed in the social and institutional arrangements that already exist. As a result, they will generally be expected to navigate among their various values and commitments within, rather than apart from, modern medicine. Nevertheless, the practices of prayer, baptism, and Eucharist can lead to transformative practices at the end of life.

Drawing closer and closer to death—a process, we do well to remember, that occurs throughout our lives—those shaped by these Christian practices will be accustomed to giving over their life to God. They did so in their baptism. They were formed into the broken body of Jesus, the one who gave himself for all humanity, through the Eucharist. They witnessed the encounter of the gospel with death through the proclamation of the word of life. The burden of agency will not finally be solved or taken away but can be experienced differently once our underlying assumptions about human agency are challenged by an alternative vision. Infused with Christian language and formed by Christian practices, dying can become a culmination and extension of a lifelong process of entrusting one's life and future to the God who is Lord over both life and death.

Conclusion

Humanity Sub Specie Mortis

Narratives have the power to form and shape our moral imagination in ways that arguments often cannot. In this conclusion, rather than simply recount the argument, I want to demonstrate its significance through a series of stories. The three stories I will tell shaped my own moral imagination in a crucial period of my own life. As mentioned in the introduction to this book, on my first day of my doctoral program, I was diagnosed with cancer. To be sure, my cancer did not carry a terminal diagnosis, but it did require treatment through surgery and chemotherapy. It was a major life experience for me and my wife, both because of the disruption of our "normal" lives and because of the threat it seemed to pose to our ability to have children in the future, a desire we shared. Despite all the challenges, it was important for me to carry on with my life and work, which meant that I would teach bioethics to undergraduate discussion sections Friday afternoons and then walk five blocks to the hospital to receive my weekly injection of healing poisons (otherwise known as bleomycin, etoposide, and cisplatin).

It was during this time that I first began to reckon with some of the deeper themes of this book. I began to recognize that being an embodied person in a finite and fallen world means that I am vulnerable (shocker, I know). I saw that my habitual way of thinking (or not thinking) about ability and disability was based on the assumption that I would always be able bodied. I now recognized this as a lie; each of us is always only temporarily able bodied. Therefore, each person must at some point reckon with their limitedness (finitude). I began to notice that medicine, as it is commonly practiced, is often a way of ignoring or transcending limits, a fact made especially clear by the difficulty many doctors have in talking with patients about death and dying. Like most of us, doctors prefer to speak about things they can control. I also began to recognize my own imprisonment within the myth of control. Especially when cancer threatened "the five-year plan" my wife and I had for having children (i.e., once we had been married for five years), I began to realize that what I *had thought* was under my control was not, in fact, under my control in an ultimate sense. This realization has profoundly impacted my understanding of parenting in general. I also came to see death as a symbol of all that ultimately lies beyond human control.

It was also during this time that I encountered the three stories that follow. The first, a short story by agrarian author-poet-activist Wendell Berry, will bring into focus the diagnosis of the problem we have been exploring in this book—burdened agency. The second, the story of Kara Tippetts and Brittany Maynard, two women who struggled publicly with terminal cancer, highlights the two "scripts" for dying in the modern social imaginary. Finally, the story of baby Jack, who was born with Trisomy-13 and lived for two days, points to how the practices of the church can transform moral agents—in this case, Jack's parents—in such a way that they can bear burdened agency well.

BURLEY COULTER

Wendell Berry's short story "Fidelity" chronicles the peculiar death of Burley Coulter, an elderly man and member of the community (or "membership") of Port William, Kentucky, a fictional town in which many of Berry's novels and stories are set.[1] Burley Coulter was an unconventional character. He is described as a man "freely in love with freedom and with pleasures." He "watched the world with an amused, alert eye to see what it would do next, and if the world did not seem inclined to get on very soon to anything of interest, he gave it his help." Burley never settled down with a wife and family on a farm, as many of Berry's character do. Rather, he was "by calling and by devotion a man of the woods and streams. When duty did not keep him in the fields, he would be hunting or fishing or roaming about in search of herbs or wild fruit, or merely roaming about to see what he could see."

Burley had an illegitimate son, Danny Branch, through a youthful tryst with Kate Helen Branch, who remained the love of Burley's life, though they never married. While he was late in acknowledging Danny as his own, he did finally do so. Danny would call him "Uncle Burley," but the two of them loved each other like father and son. Burley was unpredictable, but he was also—and this is key—faithful. "Though he was wild, he didn't steal or lie or misrepresent himself."

One day after farming, Danny finds the elderly Burley hunched over, asleep and unresponsive in the cab of his truck. He and his cousin Nathan are concerned about Burley but conflicted about what to do. Danny wonders if they should take him to the hospital. Nathan responds, "He's never been to a doctor since I've known him. He said he wouldn't go. You going to knock him in the head before you take him?" Hannah, Nathan's wife, wonders if it might have been better for Burley to "die in his sleep out at work with us or under a tree somewhere." But he didn't, and something must be done. "So they took him. They took him because they wanted to do more for him than they could do, and they could think of nothing else. Nathan held out the longest, and he gave in only because he was uncertain." When Burley arrives at the big hospital, he is disoriented and confused. "He was no longer in his right mind, they thought, because he was no longer in his right place." Over the next few days, "Burley slipped away toward death. But the people of the hospital did not call it dying; they called it a coma. They spoke of curing him. They spoke of his recovery."

Here, we begin to see a crack opening between two worlds, which in another essay Berry would call "the world of love [and] the world of efficiency—the world, that is, of specialization, machinery, and abstract procedure."[2] As the doctor speaks "fluently from within the bright orderly enclosure of his explanation, like a man in a glass booth . . . [Burley's family] stood looking in at him from the larger, looser, darker order of their merely human love." As they listen to the doctors, "they looked at each other, and their eyes met in confusion, as if they had come to the wrong place."

The hospital is, as Berry describes it, a place of profound alienation, filled with "strange, resistant objects." In a key scene, Burley's company returns to the hospital "to enact again the strange rite of offering themselves where they could not be received." Berry is worth quoting at length.

When they returned on yet another visit and found the old body still as it had been, a mere passive addition to the complicated machines that kept it minimally alive, they saw finally that in their attempt to help they had not helped but only complicated his disease beyond their power to help. And they thought with regret of the time when the thing that was wrong with him had been simply unknown, and there had been only it and him and him and them in the place they had known together. Loving him, wanting to help him, they had given him over to "the best of modern medical care"—which meant, as they now saw, that they had abandoned him.

At this point in the story, things take an unexpected turn when Danny decides he can no longer abide such a situation. In the dead of night, he leaves his house, telling his wife only that "if somebody wants to know, I said something about Indiana." With that, he drives his beaten-down truck along "the succession of ever wider and faster roads that led to the seasonless, sunless, and moonless world where Burley lay in his bonds." Sneaking into the hospital, he cuts Burley's medical tubes, places him on a gurney, covers him with a sheet and wheels him right out the door.

The rest of the narrative follows two storylines: on the one hand, it follows Danny as he takes Burley to the abandoned and overgrown "Old Barn" in Stepstone Hollow, a familiar place where the two of them regularly rested during long hunting trips. There, Danny lovingly prepares a place for burial while Burley slowly fades into death. When Danny finally laid Burley into the stone casket (made from river rock) lining the grave, the author evokes themes of submissive receptivity: "[Danny] stepped into the grave and laid the body down. He composed it like a sleeper, laying the hands together as before. And the body seemed to accept again its stillness and its deep sleep, submissive to the motion of the world until the world's end."

The other storyline follows Detective Kyle Bode, who arrives in Port William looking to solve the case of the missing "old geezer" and his "kidnapper," whom he is certain is "this damned redneck, Danny Branch." Bode's character is a counterpart and foil to the ethos and value system of Danny, Burley, and the whole Port William "membership." A generation ago, Bode's father had escaped from "Nowhere" Kentucky to the city of Louisville, where he had become a successful dealer in farm equipment (not an admirable role in Berry's moral universe). Bode himself escaped the fate of inheriting the dealership, feeling that farmers and their ilk were "beneath" him. Bode is dilettantish, "sexually liberated," insecure, and perpetually dissatisfied.

As Bode talks with Henry Catlett, the family's friend and lawyer, he speculates as to the possible motive for the kidnapping. "It's a crime involving the new medical technology. I mean, some of this stuff is unheard of. We're living in the future right now. I figure this crime is partly motivated by anxiety about this new stuff. Like maybe the guy that did it is some kind of religious nut." That, or he's angling for an early inheritance.

I do not want to spoil the end of the story, so I will not reveal how these two storylines eventually intersect into a fitting conclusion. Instead, I want to use the story to review a central theme of this book—namely, agency in dying. This book approaches this issue from the vantage point of modern practices of dying. For it is the practical problem of "dying well" that has become an existential issue for a great many people in modern society. In "Fidelity," we see that the problem of a good death for Burley Coulter has been complicated by a medical culture that, once initiated, drives him and his family deeper and deeper into the logic of the hospital. They are experiencing what I have called burdened agency. On the one hand, they have a burden *of* agency, which is to say that Burley's death is marked by a proliferation of choice—choices about whether to bring Burley to the hospital, choices about what sorts of treatments to subject him to, choices about how far is too far. Having brought Burley into the hospital, they would soon be expected to make concrete choices about the manner and timing of his death—choices forestalled by Danny's decisive choice to bring Burley home. The doctor represents the stance of "technological brinkmanship," the desire to come as close to the line of overtreatment as possible without crossing it. As is clear from the language of the story, the greatest threat to a good death, for Berry at least, involves the near certainty of overmedicalization in the ICU.

Choice, of course, is not inherently bad. To speak of the burden *of* agency is not to conclude that it would be better if choices were withheld from patients at the end of life. The language of burdening refers rather to the phenomenological level, the experience of *having* to choose. These choices may feel especially burdensome when they arise for the very first time when someone is in the process of dying. Berry's story was published in the earlier 1990s, likely written some time before. At that time, the medicalization of dying was rapidly increasing, and palliative medicine and hospice had not yet become mainstream. In a contemporary retelling, perhaps Uncle Burley would have had a living will that could guide the doctors, or the family may have had end-of-life discussions. Perhaps these could relieve some of the burden of agency. But as Berry notes in another essay, medicine expects patients to make an autonomous choice on matters that are beyond them.

> An "informed decision" is really not even imaginable for most medical patients and their families, who have no competent understanding of either the patient's illness or the recommended medical or surgical procedure. Moreover, patients and their families are not likely to know the doctor, the surgeon, or any of the other people on whom the patient's life will depend. In the hospital, [patients and proxies] are more than likely to be proceeding entirely upon faith—and this is a peculiar and scary faith, for it must be placed not in a god but in mere people, mere procedures, mere chemicals, and mere machines.[3]

But it is not simply the existence of choices that burdens agency. At the same time we are burdened with choices, we are also less able to rely on cultural guidance about *how* to choose wisely and well. This leads to a loss of cultural aptitude and an increasing sense of awkwardness about speaking about death or speaking with those who are grieving. In "Fidelity," this quality is, importantly, most clearly embodied by the doctors and by Detective Bode, who is a thoroughly "modern" kind of figure in comparison with the rest of the Port William membership. Although not especially (or, at least, ostentatiously) religious, Danny and the rest belong to a stronger culture, rooted in a particular sense of community and a particular relationship with the land. At times, they exhibit the familiar simplicity toward death that Philippe Ariès spoke about, as we see in Berry's account of Burley's actual moment of death.

> On one of these trips to the barn, [Danny] knew as he entered the doorway that the breaths had stopped, and he stopped, and then went soundlessly in where the body lay. It looked unaccountably small. Now of its long life in this place there remained only this small artifact of flesh

and bone. In the hospital, Burley's body had seemed to Danny to be off in another world; he had not been able to rid himself of the feeling that he was looking at it through a lens or a window. Here, the old body seemed to belong to this world absolutely, it was so accepting now of all that had come to it, even its death. Burley had died as he had slept—he had not moved. Danny leaned and picked up the still hands and laid them together. He went back to his digging and worked on as before.

When I first encountered this story, I remember thinking that there was something right about what Danny had done. Some of us more urbane readers may be uncomfortable with Burley's dying unceremoniously in an old barn in the woods, but it was a *fitting* death, given who Burley was. The rightness of the death, however, is not simply a matter of authenticity, of Burley dying *on his own terms*. Rather, it involves Burley being restored to his place and his people. It also involves Danny drawing on the customs and forms of life he had inherited to accompany his father into death and to face it with equanimity.

BRITTANY AND KARA

One day, around this same time, I also heard the moving story of Brittany Maynard, the twenty-nine-year-old California woman who had moved to Oregon to take advantage of the Death with Dignity law in that state. Given my own diagnosis and the direction my research interests were taking, I read her account of her decision (published by CNN) with interest. Brittany had a rare form of inoperable and incurable brain cancer, which caused her to have intense headaches and seizures. She knew the only option for treatment—full-brain radiation—would come with unacceptable side effects and would not cure her but only, perhaps, extend her life while sacrificing its quality. She explained why she did not see hospice care as an option: "Even with palliative medication, I could develop potentially morphine-resistant pain and suffer personality changes and verbal, cognitive and motor loss of virtually any kind. Because the rest of my body is young and healthy, I am likely to physically hang on for a long time even though cancer is eating my mind. I probably would have suffered in hospice care for weeks or even months. And my family would have had to watch that."[4] In Brittany's mind, this would be a "nightmare scenario."

I also read with interest her impassioned defense of "death with dignity" legislation. She explained the hoops and barriers she faced in gaining access. She explained that seeking the drugs did not make her "suicidal." "I do not want to die. But I am dying. And I want to die on my own terms." She explained the "tremendous sense of relief" and "peace" she has gained from the sense of control the prescription gives her, describing it as a "safety net." She questioned the right of anyone to deny her what she sees as her own right of self-determination. And she ended with a plea for expanded access. "When my suffering becomes too great, I can say to all those I love, 'I love you; come be by my side, and come say goodbye as I pass into whatever's next.' I will die upstairs in my bedroom with my husband, mother, stepfather and best friend by my side and pass peacefully. I can't imagine trying to rob anyone else of that choice." Brittany's story immediately struck a nerve and sparked a national conversation about end-of-life options. In public interviews and documentary films, Brittany offered her story, which became a rallying cry for proponents of assisted suicide/medical assistance in dying.

In a memoir, written by Brittany's mother, Deborah Ziegler, we get an even more intimate picture of Brittany's story than in her public statements and interviews.[5] The book is vulnerable and touching. A sympathetic reader (especially a parent) cannot help but be moved by it. I was especially curious about what a mother's account might reveal about how Brittany's ethical values came to be formed, about what her experience of the medical system involved, and about whether she, or anyone around her, ever had any doubts about her desire for assisted dying. Of course, it can be dangerous to play the role of armchair psychoanalyst, reducing a complex inner life into a set of interpretive categories that, by the very nature of the case, cannot capture that person in their entirety. I want to be sensitive to this truth. At the same time, we *can* learn from other people's stories. Since this book is about the nature of moral agency at the end of life, Brittany's story—which tapped so powerfully into a broader cultural current—helps us to see aspects of what we have called the modern social imaginary.

Ziegler's account of her daughter's diagnosis and initial treatment reveals a highly ambivalent relationship with medicine and medical culture. She expresses outrage and frustration about an early appointment ending in the doctor dismissing Brittany as having stress-related "women's headaches," rather than ordering a scan that might have caught the cancer earlier. When Ziegler arrived to see Brittany during her next hospital visit, Brittany was unconscious, likely suffering from an overdose of Dilaudid, which required Narcan to stabilize. It turns out Brittany was especially sensitive to this powerful pain-relieving drug. Ziegler spends time "trying to determine if the nurse was someone who could be trusted around my child." She tells of doctors consistently "avoiding eye contact" and talking *around* the diagnosis: rather than a "tumor," it's "a large infiltrating nonenhancing lesion present in the left prefrontal lobe, and it extends posteriorly into the left temporal lobe."

Within minutes of receiving her diagnosis, Brittany asked the doctor point-blank, "Do you transfer patients to Oregon?" When the doctor balked, Brittany was direct. "If you don't know why I'd want to transfer to Oregon, this discussion is over." At the same time, Ziegler, at least, held out hope for a medical cure. "Science. Medicine. They would save Brittany. Or perhaps God, through a doctor using science and medicine, would save Brittany. Yes, a combination of faith and science and medicine would be unbeatable. Or so I told myself." Brittany, however, had a bracing realism about her situation. "I'm toast, Momma. . . . I need you to get that. I have a giant tumor that is going to kill me in the most horrible fucking way if I don't do something about it. . . . This monster tumor isn't going to stop. It's going to change grades, and stage four brain cancer is cruel. I'll be paralyzed. I'll lose my memory. I might not even know who you are anymore. . . . I'll lose everything that makes me who I am." Although Brittany agreed to undergo surgery to remove a section of the tumor, she was adamantly opposed to other aggressive treatments she saw as futile. "I am not going to let them burn the shit out of my brain. I've read about radiation. . . . Cut. Poison. Burn. Everywhere we go. This is what they will say—in nicer terminology. . . . The therapy is worse than the disease. I'm not going to allow them to damage my cognitive ability. I'm not letting them destroy the quality of the little life I have left."

After her surgery, Brittany's road was rocky. She experienced intermittent depression and anger. At one low point, she descends into a possibly drug-and-cancer-induced rage, leaving her mother "hiding from the rapier-sharp edge of my daughter's tongue." At another point, when Ziegler tries to have a conversation with Brittany about faith and religion, her daughter flies off the handle, leading to a physical altercation. Ziegler conjectures that these "bouts of egocentrism and insensitivity to the needs of others" were caused by the effects of Brittany's cancer on her brain. Either that, or Brittany was trying subconsciously to "cut the cord" with her mother to make it easier to go through with her plan for assisted dying.

Despite the relational stress and challenges, the family walked the road together. They found a beautiful house to rent together in an exclusive Portland neighborhood. They made the most of their short time together, taking trips to exotic locations between doctors' visits. Brittany spent time advocating publicly for her "right to die." When it was finally time to go through with assisted dying, her mother was there by her side, along with her stepfather, her husband, and a close friend.

In Ziegler's telling, we can see the highly choreographed but also *reflexive* nature of Brittany's death. "Brittany had been very specific about how she wanted her death to be, who she wanted in the room with her, where she wanted them to be, and what she wanted to hear. Britt was especially worried that she might lose consciousness and yet be able to hear us for some time afterward. She specifically instructed us not to weep, make sad noises, or discuss her dying until everyone was sure that she had expired. She selected poems written by Mary Oliver, her favorite poet, to be read to her in the minutes after she ingested the medicine." In the end, her death was very quick. At the end of her book, Ziegler sums up her view—and Brittany's view—of assisted dying:

> The "culture of cure" has led to a fairy-tale belief that doctors can always fix our problems. We have lost sight of reality. All life ends. Death is not necessarily the enemy in all cases. Sometimes a gentle passing is a gift. Misguided doctors caught up in an aspirational belief that they must extend life, whatever the cost, cause individuals and families unnecessary suffering. Brittany stood up to bullies. She never thought anyone else had the right to tell her how long she should suffer. The right to die for the terminally ill is a human rights issue. Plain and simple.

As mentioned, Brittany's story resonated deeply with many people. But not all agreed with her pursuit of assisted dying, even if they did share her conviction that "death is not necessarily the enemy in all cases." One woman, Kara Tippetts, ventured an open letter to Brittany as an attempt to get her to see things differently. Tippetts was a thirty-eight-year-old mother of four, who was also dying of cancer (in her case, breast cancer, which had spread through her lymph nodes into her bones, major organs, and brain).[6] She was deeply moved by Brittany's story. In her open letter, she thanked Brittany for sharing her story publicly. She lamented the "hard path you are being asked to travel." She acknowledged realities of fear, pain, and suffering. But she also pressed forcefully against the "horrible lie, that your dying will not be beautiful. That the suffering will be too great." Drawing from her own Christian perspective, she noted, "Suffering is not the absence of goodness, it is not the absence of beauty, but perhaps it can be the place where true beauty can be known." She pointed to the significance of the death and resurrection of Jesus. "He overcame the death you and I are facing in our cancer. He longs to know you, to shepherd you in your dying." She offered to "jump on a plane tomorrow to meet you and share the beautiful brokenness of my story and meet you in yours if you would ever consider having me." She noted her regret at "the multitudes that are looking at your story and believing the lie that suffering is a mistake, that dying isn't to be braved." Rather, Kara suggested, "I get to partner with my doctor in my dying, and it's going to be a beautiful and painful journey for us all. But, hear me—it is not a mistake—beauty will meet us in that last breath." Getting to the heart of the matter, she explained, "There is dignity in dying and suffering even if she does it without taking this pill. . . . She can live a dignified life in that doctors who care about her dying can comfort her and walk with her in her dying so she does die with dignity in the moment she's called to die."

In an interview, Kara explained how Christian faith and practice prepared her to approach death in this way:

> When I speak, I often tell people who are in a season of being healthy, "Are you a student of your faith? Are you being mentored? Are you growing near to Jesus in ways that will carry you if you get a story like mine eventually?" And so, I feel like my years up to now have been spent being that—being a student of my faith, being mentored as much as I could, and knowing God's Word. So now, as it's hard for me to read, it's hard for me to have time with a mentor, the energy I spent then is what carries me now. As I've been asked to receive this story, God was gracious to grow me to where He did before the story came.[7]

This changed the way Kara viewed her own cancer. "Cancer was this gift that exposed us to what is important and what's valuable, parenting with kindness, loving your husband, living well." That's not to say that all is rosy. For example, her illness posed a threat to her own sense of identity. "Who am I without hair? Without breasts? Without a uterus? Do I still have value?" She notes that chemotherapy caused early menopause so that she went from feeling like a thirty-year-old to feeling like an eighty-year-old in a matter of months. She acknowledges her anger about having to die. "I feel like I'm a little girl at a party whose dad is asking her to leave early, and I am throwing a fit. I'm not afraid of dying. I just don't want to go." At the same time, her suffering also points her toward deeper truths. In speaking about her transition from therapeutic treatments to hospice care, Kara confesses,

> I just want to be strong, but that's not in the cards for me right now. So, when you see your weakness, it can be discouraging. I let myself be discouraged. I let myself be sad. I think it's part of being authentic and real in this, that it's not all easy, and that's okay. And it shows me that I'm needy. And when you're needy, you're needy for something. And I'm so needy for Jesus to help me, walk with me through these last days, these last moments. And so, when I see that neediness, I am not discouraged.

I have suggested that particular substantive beliefs about human selfhood and moral agency are embedded within our institutions, discourses, and practices of dying. These beliefs and assumptions often remain subterranean and inarticulate, but this fact does not make them any less powerful and persuasive. Indeed, the strength of a set of norms is often directly correlated with the degree to which those norms are taken for granted. In other words, substantive beliefs and assumptions about human personhood and moral agency constitute a "social imaginary" that sets the terms for how we die.

In Brittany's and Kara's stories, we see two people approaching death along the lines of the "cultural scripts for dying" (Banner) explored in chapter 2 of this book. These scripts have each increasingly entered the mainstream as our society seeks to enable people to die in ways that are more humane and that do not simply extend the dying process (and the suffering of dying) through technological brinkmanship. Brittany's story, especially, reflects Charles Taylor's account of the "modern identity" insofar as it demonstrates a commitment to the values of autonomy and control, avoidance of suffering, and the expression of individuality and authenticity. Kara's story does not deny these goods but subordinates them within a different sort of "social imaginary," one that sees dependence, weakness, and vulnerability as part of the human experience and that has been conditioned to see such things as the place where God's grace can be experienced through an identification with Christ, the suffering one.

These two stories, read in juxtaposition with each other, bring up the matter of the ethics of euthanasia and assisted suicide. In introducing the two scripts, I noted a set of shortcomings for each, along with pitfalls shared by both (such as their mutual inapplicability to the prolonged-dwindling illness trajectory and their overreliance on a particular notion of the relationship between freedom of choice and personal identity). One should not imagine, however, that the subsequent philosophical and theological analysis aims to present each script on an equal footing; the general tone of the analysis quite obviously favors the latter over the former. The discussion about hospice generally has regarded *how best* to conceptualize its practice; the discussion about physician-assisted suicide (PAS) and euthanasia has tended to focus on *whether* such practices should be considered illicit or should be made more readily available to individuals at the end of life.

For all of this, I have not ventured a conclusive judgment about whether PAS and euthanasia should be considered morally wrong or morally acceptable. One reason for reticence on this issue is the fact that individual cases admit of much more complexity than can be considered in a more general discussion. Another reason is that this book has primarily focused on "attitudes" and "postures" toward agency in dying from a single, tradition-specific perspective. It is not entirely clear to me how an analysis on this level would yield a general conclusion about PAS and euthanasia with universal moral applicability. However, the particular posture outlined here does, I believe, correspond with the practices of hospice medicine and palliative care in a way that is not true for assisted dying. In hospice, dying can be understood as a kenotic act of dispossession and witness that occurs when one is able to surrender oneself to a death that is inevitable and (ultimately) out of one's control. Describing assisted suicide in this way would be tendentious (as noted before, maintaining control is the central concern of most PAS patients).

How a community that is formed by the Christian standpoint—as articulated in this book—would evaluate particular instances of PAS and euthanasia or how it would go about formulating a position regarding law and public policy is open to further discussion. I would strongly urge hesitation with regard to legalization of these practices but for reasons that have more to do with prudential judgment about the protection of vulnerable individuals and concerns about the erosion of the guiding moral ideals of the profession of medicine.

The question of how best to meet a friend in her pain and suffering is a complicated one. But by and large, I suggest in all humility that it would be better and more fitting not to eliminate the sufferer in the name of eliminating suffering. I am reminded here of the ancient story of Job, that prototypical sufferer. Job experienced total pain. He had immense physical, emotional, and spiritual suffering. He had painful boils. He lost his children and much of his wealth. In many ways, he was a shell of his former self. At the beginning of his story, we see two sets of reactions to his condition. One comes from his wife, the other from his friends. His wife, who we must remember has also suffered greatly, exclaims desperately, "Are you still trying to maintain your integrity? Curse God and die!" (Job 2:9). We need not denigrate her, as some commentators do, as an unfaithful and wicked wife. Indeed, she seems to be expressing the very understandable emotions of an agonized caregiver. Nevertheless, her response can be contrasted with the response of Job's friends. "When three of Job's friends heard of the tragedy he had suffered, they got together and traveled from their homes to comfort and console him. . . . Wailing loudly, they tore their robes and threw dust into the air over their heads to show their grief. Then they sat on the ground with him for seven days and nights. No one said a word to Job, for they saw that his suffering was too great for words" (Job 2:11–13). Unfortunately, eventually the friends start talking, and when they do, they are much less helpful to Job. But at least initially, they seem to have done something right in expressing solidarity through mere presence. They would rather be present in his pain than see him end his pain by ending his life. The intuitive public appeal of assisted dying is, at least in part, a reflection on our collective failure to meet the basic needs of dying persons, including social, spiritual, and emotional needs. Dying well should not be conceived as a heroic, individualistic task. Rather, each of us can only bear the suffering of dying insofar as we are upheld by others who are willing to "bear one another's burdens, and so fulfill the law of Christ" (Gal 6:2), the one who shows us how to bear the burden of death to the very end.

BABY JACK

The final story hits a bit closer to home. Again, around this same time, I heard from two childhood friends, Scott and Meg, who were now married and expecting a child. They reached out by email to request prayer. Scott wrote, "Today's appointment was devastating and heartbreaking. All indications at this time are that our baby boy has a severe chromosomal disorder that will impact viability of his life. . . . We're not quite sure what to ask you to pray for at this point. . . . We know [God] is good, always and forever. Harder to say that now than most days, but we believe it."[8] Two days later, Meg wrote, "We received confirmation today that our baby boy (baby "JAK" as we have been calling him) has Trisomy 13. I have truly felt a supernatural peace in the past week as the Lord is breaking our hearts and giving us a deeper understanding of his mercy and joy. The next 4 months and beyond will be difficult as we cherish time with our son and pray for God to move. We don't know what is to come, but we do know that God is not surprised by this. He has gone before us and will be with us; we will not be afraid or discouraged. Deut 31:8."[9]

The emails, while communicating the essential facts, left out much of these grieving parents' experience. Speaking with them later, I began to get a fuller picture. The twenty-week ultrasound had revealed some potential issues, but Scott and Meg had not initially realized the extent of Jack's medical condition. The ultrasound techs were reticent about details and, unhelpfully in retrospect, had downplayed the results. But when the physician walked in for the follow-up, his demeanor ended any expectations that Scott and Meg were facing a minor medical issue. This was "the hardest day. . . . The rug [was] pulled out from under [us]; all [our] expectations [were] shattered."

This was also the meeting that ushered these expectant parents into the vortex of medical decision making. The doctor methodically reviewed the results of the ultrasound. He described the main issues (cleft palate, swapped organs, a defective aortic arch), noting that any one of these issues would present serious medical challenges; all of them together suggested a diagnosis "not compatible with life." From this point forward, Scott and Meg would have to negotiate a series of choices related to Meg's pregnancy and Jack's care for which they were not prepared. "I had no competence in this area; I felt totally useless and hopeless" after that initial conversation, said Meg. The doctor recommended they consider termination, adding that they needed to be aware that this option would not be available long due to local abortion laws and the stage of the pregnancy. He noted that Jack would not likely survive to full term and through the process of birth (they were reminded of these facts multiple times over the first weeks after Jack's diagnosis).

The philosopher Iris Murdoch once wrote, "At crucial moments of choice, most of the business of choosing is already over."[10] In the end, the question of whether to try to carry Jack to term wasn't much of a question because of how Scott and Meg's moral vision had been shaped by Christian faith and practices. "We confirmed whether my health was in danger and it was not, and there seemed to be no increased risk to carrying [the pregnancy] other than [the emotional risk of] personal attachment." For Scott and Meg, this settled the question about a possible termination. They would welcome this newone into their lives.[11] This decision rested for them on the "founding principle . . . that we are made in God's image. Ultimately, there was freedom and peace in knowing it *wasn't* my decision to terminate this life. That actually takes pressure off that this life is in the hands of the Lord. . . . Rather than "this is my body" and "this is a parasite" (in one extreme), or just "this is my body and I have the right to choose," [it's] this is a life that we get to steward and to parent whatever that looks like. Once that decision is off the table, it kind of narrows and simplifies the focus: this is a life, this is a child, this is our child and I am a mother, this is our first baby boy."[12] In her carefully written birth plan, Meg would later inform the care team, "Our beloved baby Jack has been diagnosed with Trisomy 13. However imperfect he appears, he is our son, whom we love deeply. This love compels us to treasure every moment of our baby's life to its fullest extent."[13]

This does not mean that matters were simple for Scott and Meg. They were still thrust into deep and complicated grief, simultaneously trying to celebrate Jack's new life while mourning having to let him go. All the while, the "rest of the world keeps going on." Meg noted how isolating this experience was and how it required "major compartmentalization for survival," especially as she returned to work. It was emotionally jarring. "In the same day I was emailing about funeral plans for my son, we had birthing class together.... We could *not* mention what we were going through."[14]

I asked Meg how she managed this tension between grief and celebration. It was difficult for her to explain. "I remember sitting in the parking lot ... waiting to go back in[to the hospital], having the oddest sense ... that I felt blessed. I had that sense from the Lord that I was blessed. Still sadness and confusion but peace. And also, clearly, that doesn't make sense in that moment to say I am blessed.... [It] was not logical or reasonable, which is part of how we knew it was from the Lord. Since then, we have seen a lot of ways we *have* been blessed."[15]

Jack was born in the early morning hours on March 6, 2014, 6 lb 12 oz, complete with a full head of hair. "Grey and gooey and beautiful."[16] Jack had six fingers on each hand, which he memorably held out in a "shaka" pose (the image of his hand would be emblazoned on merchandise for the family's charitable organization, "Jack's Aloha"). Initial assessments confirmed for Scott and Meg that attempting a major surgery would not likely extend Jack's life span or increase his quality of life considerably. They decided on comfort care to better cherish their short time with him. Over a very full two and a half days, their area of the children's hospital became something of a spectacle, as uncles and aunts, grandparents, and friends came together around Jack and his parents. A pastor "came in to pray over [Jack] and dedicate [him] to the Lord" with anointing oil. Scott and Meg's attitude was, "We want him dedicated, we want worship, my family will bring instruments and we will sing, and we will model celebration, even for the medical staff." In normal circumstances, this may have been an unacceptable interruption to the regimented and antiseptic order of the hospital, but the medical staff made exceptions to the rules for Jack's case. "Meg's family is fairly comfortable with boundary-pushing," Scott told me with a grin.

Because of the issue with his heart, Scott and Meg knew Jack would not live very long. He died surrounded by a community of love and care. In a journal entry, Meg wrote, "With angels in the room, we sang for the Holy Spirit to come. I sang to the Lord that we *surrendered* you to Him, you were a precious gift.... We all sang praises and I couldn't stop kissing you. We sang as a family and you were calm and serene and stable.... We held you and kissed your hand. Your heartrate finally stopped as you peacefully breathed your last breath on earth and your first with your Heavenly Father."[17]

The theme of surrender is prominent in Scott and Meg's story. "If we think that God is allowing this to happen for whatever reason . . . then [the question becomes] 'how do we surrender?'"[18] When I asked them how they learned to surrender, they mentioned prayer and fasting, among other spiritual disciplines like communal worship. "It's a combination of things. Prayer life . . . in context with a lot of other things that have informed and grown our prayer life. . . . As we have grown in enjoyment of worship—to worship a God and sing and be reminded of who I am singing to—it continues to shape your belief so that entering into prayer . . . I can pray boldly, and confidently, and know I will not be abandoned."[19] Regarding fasting, Scott noted, "To deny myself creates space to pursue the Lord, while preparing myself for times when I will be denied [things]. So when I pray, I can turn fully to the Lord and desire what he has for me."[20]

This echoes the themes explored in the preceding chapters. In these responses, there is something of the "spirituality of martyrdom," which becomes a "witness" to Christ in and through a free giving-up of the self even in the face of death (in this case, the death of a dear son and the death of a dream of a particular vision of parenthood). There is also an acceptance of creaturely finitude, a recognition that each life is a unique, never-to-be-repeated opportunity with a genuine beginning and end. This helped them to see and accept Jack's existence as a gift, a life to be respected and received with gratitude.

It is true that death limits one's life. But as Barth reminds us, there is a limit also to death: God is Lord over life *and* death. For Scott and Meg, this truth became clearer to them as they contemplated the nature of heaven. "Under [our] prayer life is the actual faith in God. . . . We grieve differently as those with hope, not as those without hope. Prayer is the manifestation of the faith . . . and prayer is what brings that to life practically."[21] As they contemplate what is beyond this life, knowing the reward of what's next makes this life "grown strangely dim." This has taught them to "fear death less," sometimes "even bordering on looking forward to it." But theirs is not simply an otherworldly faith. Jack's death "spurred a bit of urgency as well—the desire to bring heaven here . . . has helped [them] to see how much time matters here."[22] This is an expression of the dual movement of the Lord's Prayer, discussed in the previous chapter. "Thy Kingdom come; Thy will be done on earth as it is in heaven." As Sarah Coakley reminds us, this prayer is emblematic of all Christian prayer in being simultaneously a movement of *unselfing* (*Thy* will be done) and an orientation of submissive receptivity toward God (*Thy* will be done on earth as it is in heaven). This culminates in an ethic of dispossession—a willingness to be let go, to be vulnerable before God and others. This is possible, Stanley Hauerwas reminds us, only through trusting faith that ultimately the goal of life is neither control nor is it "to get out of life alive" but rather simply to trust in the one who has already triumphed over the principalities and powers.

Jack's story became a powerful witness to Scott and Meg's community, including myself and my family. It demonstrated the falsity of the worldly perspective that a life such as Jack's is meaningless or simply involves meaningless suffering. Part of the challenge of burdened agency is in how it places individuals in a position of feeling as though they must grapple with and decide about ultimate realities. If meaning is to be found, one must forge one's own meaning in the face of a fragmented world. Jack's life reminds us that it's not up to us to determine what can or can't be meaningful. From the Christian standpoint, the goal is to learn to receive such things as meaning and purpose from the Lord. Christian practices like prayer, worship, and fasting inculcate a receptive form of agency before God. A person formed by such practices is taught, implicitly and explicitly, to hold such an attitude even in the face of death.

At Jack's memorial service, Scott spoke eloquently about the meaning of Jack's life. I will give him the last word.

As I put my pen down and looked back at the words, it became easier to see the beauty and power of Jack's adventure. The job of parents is to teach their children, but for me, it was Jack who taught me a powerful lesson. Jack taught me the importance of living a life worth writing about. And I think there were two main reasons why his story was so wonderful:

His story had a purpose—We are all created for something. And as we live, we are all betting on something. What is it that I am betting on? Myself? Our days are too short to waste them being self-centered. Material goods? Our days are too short to be chasing things that rust or fade—things you can't take with you when you're dead. Jack reminded me of the importance of considering our legacies. How can we invest our time and gifts in a way that has lasting impact? How can we set our minds on something outside of and greater than ourselves?

His story was lived in community—I looked at who he was surrounded by, not just in the hospital but really for all 9 months—family and friends that loved him dearly, that encouraged him, that laughed and cried with him, and that prayed for him from afar—and I ask myself—who am I surrounding myself with? We were created to be in community, and life is far sweeter being surrounded by people. It's not always easy—in fact, it's often messy—but it is those times of trial where relationships are forged. Think of iron—you can't just lean two pieces together to bind them. You have to put them into the fire. But as I said, in community is where life and love are found.

So, as we wake up each day and strive to be purposeful and in community, our stories will take on new life. And as for Jack, I am so thankful that with his legacy of purpose and community comes an eternity with Jesus, as his story has only just begun. I close with a snippet from C. S. Lewis, who as usual says it best. This is from his book *The Last Battle*—"All his life and all his adventure had only been the cover and the title page—now at last he begins the great story—which goes on forever, in which every chapter is better than the one before."

Amen.

Notes

INTRODUCTION. The Landscape of Modern Dying

1. McGill, *Death and Life*, 26.
2. Gawande, *Being Mortal*.
3. See Nussbaum, *The Finest Traditions of My Calling*.
4. This book does not draw a strong distinction between "theology" and "religion." Although the common convention of distinguishing the "descriptive" study of religion from the "normative" study of theology has some utility, it is not entirely satisfying in practice. Neither is the assumption that the study of religion occurs from an "outsider" perspective and the study of theology occurs from an "insider" perspective. In this book, a closer analogy for the distinction between "theology" and "religion" can be found in the categories of "theory" and "practice," if the latter terms are immediately qualified by a recognition of their constant interrelation and the fluidity of their boundaries. Religious practices are lived articulations of theological concepts, just as theological concepts are worked out and revised in the lived reality of religious practices. Religion is implicit theology; theology is explicit religion. For an immensely helpful (and entertaining) account that questions rigid distinctions between these categories, see Rogers, "Theology in the Curriculum of a Secular Religious Studies Department."

ONE. Burdened Agency

1. Kierkegaard, "At a Graveside," 91. Portions of this chapter were originally published in my article, "The Phenomenon of Burdened Agency."
2. This story is adapted from Byock, *Dying Well*, 26–27.

3. See Hafner, "In Ill Doctor." The quotations in the following two paragraphs are also from this article.

4. Clinicians and ethicists vigorously debate the best terminology to describe what has traditionally been called physician-assisted suicide. Many advocates prefer terms such as "medical aid in dying" (MAID) or "physician assistance in hastening death" out of a concern to avoid a description that entails negative ethical evaluation from the outset. This is a valid concern. In my judgment, however, the proposed terminological changes occlude the moral issue rather than clarify it. The language of "suicide" makes clear that the death is willed *and enacted* by the patient herself. MAID, on the other hand, is already being used (in Canada at the time of writing) to refer to a broader set of actions that also includes active euthanasia administered by physicians. For this reason, I tend to use the term "physician-assisted suicide," but I am not dogmatic about this choice.

5. See Pereira, "Legalizing Euthanasia or Assisted Suicide."

6. The terms "modernity," "advanced modernity," and other cognates do not refer to a specific time period but to a particular type of social order whose cultural ideals and institutions are marked by the rise of (a) functional rationality, (b) cultural pluralism, and (c) the dichotomy between "public" and "private" spheres of life. There is no single "modernity" but "multiple modernities" (globally) and diverse experiences of modernity (locally). I will accordingly limit myself to speaking about Western (in particular, North Atlantic) societies.

7. See, for example, Buchbinder, *Scripting Death*, especially chap. 5, "Access and the Power to Choose."

8. See, for example, Townes, *Breaking the Fine Rain of Death* and the work of Keith Wailoo, including Wailoo, *Dying in the City of the Blues*, Wailoo, *How Cancer Crossed the Color Line*, Wailoo, *Drawing Blood*, and Wailoo and Pemberton, *The Troubled Dream of Genetic Medicine*.

9. See Soto, Martin, and Gong, "Healthcare Disparities in Critical Illness"; Mantwill, Monestel-Umaña, and Schulz, "The Relationship between Health Literacy and Health Disparities"; Williams and Jackson, "Social Sources of Racial Disparities in Health"; and Dunlop et al., "Gender and Ethnic/Racial Disparities."

10. See Kaufman, *Ordinary Medicine*.

11. Tessman, *Burdened Virtues*, 4.

12. Tessman, *Burdened Virtues*, 8.

13. Tessman, *Burdened Virtues*, 12.

14. Nuland, *How We Die*, 254.

15. The two realms, what we might call the material and the ideal, exist in dialectical relationship in which each influences the other. An analysis of the modern experience of dying should include attention to both structural and cultural realities.

The current chapter focuses primarily on the material realm and the following chapter focuses primarily on the ideal, but the two should be read together as an interrelated analysis of the same phenomenon.

16. Quoting J. Guitton, in Ariès, *The Hour of Our Death*, 10.
17. Ariès, *The Hour of Our Death*, 18.
18. Green, *Beyond the Good Death*, 5.
19. Callahan, *The Troubled Dream of Life*, 33.
20. Ariès, *The Hour of Our Death*, 18–19.
21. Ariès, *The Hour of Our Death*, 18.
22. For two notable recent attempts to reclaim the wisdom of the *ars moriendi* tradition for modern health care, see Dugdale, *The Lost Art of Dying* and Verhey, *The Christian Art of Dying*.
23. Green, *Beyond the Good Death*, 6. There is, however, an irony here, which has not been widely acknowledged. For, as Charles Taylor notes, in this highly choreographed and social script is reflected a spirituality of death that arose in early medieval European society and was reinforced by mendicant preaching. This new stance emphasized the deathbed as the scene of individual judgment and therefore represented "both a Christianization, and an individuation" of dying. The implication is that the practices of dying in this premodern age contained the seeds for its eventual erosion. See Taylor, *A Secular Age*, 65–70.
24. Ariès, *The Hour of Our Death*, 11.
25. Berry, *The Art of the Commonplace*.
26. Reiser, *Medicine and the Reign of Technology*, 20.
27. Nuland, *How We Die*, 254.
28. Reiser, *Medicine and the Reign of Technology*, 121.
29. Bishop, *The Anticipatory Corpse*, 15.
30. Foucault's account of the movement from traditional medicine to "anatomo-pathological" medicine closely tracks Reiser's account above.
31. Bishop, *The Anticipatory Corpse*, 55; emphasis added.
32. Bishop, *The Anticipatory Corpse*, 21.
33. Bishop, *The Anticipatory Corpse*, 24.
34. Callahan, *The Troubled Dream of Life*, 40–41; emphasis original.
35. Bishop, *The Anticipatory Corpse*, 25; emphasis added.
36. Green, *Beyond the Good Death*, 48.
37. Kaufman, *And a Time to Die*, 59. Quoted in Green, *Beyond the Good Death*, 66; emphasis added. One study found that 90 percent of deaths in the ICU were preceded by a decision on the part of the patient or surrogate to withhold or withdraw treatment. See Pendergast and Luce, "Increasing Incidence of Withholding and Withdrawal of Life Support."

38. Risse, *Mending Bodies, Saving Souls*, 5.

39. Gorer, "The Pornography of Death." This article was originally published in 1955. Of course, Tolstoy's haunting portrayal of *The Death of Ivan Ilyich* demonstrates that the tendency to remain silent about death was common at least as early as the 1870s.

40. Fitts and Ravdin, "What Philadelphia Physicians Tell Patients."

41. Quoted in Burt, *Death Is That Man Taking Names*, 109.

42. See, for example, The et al., "Collusion in Doctor-Patient Communication"; Drought and Koenig, "'Choice' in End-of-Life Decision Making"; and Hancock et al., "Truth Telling in Discussing."

43. Giddens, *Modernity and Self-Identity*, 244.

44. Giddens, *Modernity and Self-Identity*, 8.

45. Mitford, *The American Way of Death*; Feifel, *The Meaning of Death*; Kübler-Ross, *On Death and Dying*; Elias, *The Loneliness of the Dying*; Becker, *The Denial of Death*; Choron, *Death and Western Thought*. For the history of the death awareness movement, see Bregman, *Beyond Silence and Denial* and Doka, "The Death Awareness Movement."

46. See, for example, Gawande, "Letting Go"; Gawande, *Being Mortal*; Kalanithi, *When Breath Becomes Air*; Hitchens, *Mortality*; Didion, *The Year of Magical Thinking*; and Didion, *Blue Nights*.

47. For more, see www.deathcafe.com. In the first three years of existence, there have already been over 1,400 death cafés in twenty-six different countries. See Elmhurst, "Take Me to the Death Café."

48. Hockey, *Experiences of Death*.

49. Illich, *Medical Nemesis*, 211.

50. According to Robert Bellah, the prematurity of human birth is linked to (a) the fact of bipedalism, which constricts the mother's birth canal and (b) the link between increasing brain size and the advent of a diet of fruit and meat, occurring early in evolutionary history. For a fascinating account of how the prematurity of human birth lies at the basis of all sociality, see Bellah, *Religion in Human Evolution*, especially 122.

51. Berger and Luckmann, *The Social Construction of Reality*, 15.

52. Berger and Luckmann, *The Social Construction of Reality*, 51.

53. Giddens, *Modernity and Self-Identity*, 36.

54. Giddens, *Modernity and Self-Identity*, 35.

55. Giddens, *Modernity and Self-Identity*, 47.

56. The quotations in this paragraph are from Berger, *The Sacred Canopy*, 51, 22–23, 43–44, 12. Emphasis original.

57. See Becker, *The Denial of Death*.

58. Hannah Arendt pointed to a similar dynamic in ancient Greek conceptions of "work" and "political action," each of which seeks a level of heroic immortality that transcends the fragility of human life. See *The Human Condition*, especially chaps. 4 and 5. The problem, of course, is that each of these systems, being products of human culture, are similarly fragile and contingent. Anything, then, that threatens the favored "immortality system" is perceived as a threat to the human participant. In protecting these systems, humans are driven into conflict in a futile attempt to protect what is supposed to be invulnerable. In this regard, Augustine long ago made the observation that the fear of death (*timor mortis*) lies at the root of Rome's quest for "glory." See Dodaro, *Christ and the Just Society*, 32–43.

59. Taylor defines "subjectivation" this way: "Things that were once settled by some external reality—traditional law, say, or nature—are now referred to our choice. Issues where we were meant to accept the dictates of authority we now have to think out for ourselves." C. Taylor, *The Ethics of Authenticity*, 81.

60. As Arnold Gehlen explains, "Left in the lurch by institutions and thrown back on oneself, one can only react by taking the internal experiences which remain and exaggerating them into general validity." See Gehlen, *Anthropoligische Forschung*.

61. Giddens, *Modernity and Self-Identity*, 29.

62. Bauman, *Liquid Modernity*, 7–8. Elsewhere, Bauman spells out the existential implications of "liquid" institutional life: "Ours are the times of strongly felt moral ambiguity. These times offer us freedom of choice never before enjoyed, but also cast us into a state of uncertainty never before so agonizing. We yearn for guidance we can trust and rely upon, so that some of the haunting responsibility for our choices could be lifted from our shoulders. But the authorities we may entrust are all contested, and none seems to be powerful enough to give us the degree of reassurance we seek. In the end, we trust no authority, at least, we trust none fully, and none for long: we cannot help being suspicious about any claim to infallibility. This is the most acute and prominent practical aspect of what is justly described as the 'postmodern ethical crisis.'" See Bauman, *Postmodern Ethics*, 21.

TWO. Scripts for Dying

1. Banner, *The Ethics of Everyday Life*, 114.
2. See Putnam, *Hospice or Hemlock?*
3. Byock, Caplan, and Snyder, "Beyond Symptom Management," 57.
4. Byock, Caplan, and Snyder, "Beyond Symptom Management," 57–58; emphasis added.

5. See, for example, Quill, "Death and Dignity"; Quill, *A Midwife*, especially chaps. 7–9; Shavelson, *A Chosen Death*; Putnam, *Hospice or Hemlock?*; and Humphry, *Final Exit*.

6. See Brenan, "Americans' Strong Support for Euthanasia Persists."

7. Public Health Division, Center for Health Statistics, *Oregon Death with Dignity Act: 2022 Data Summary* (Eugene: Oregon Health Authority, 2023), https://www.oregon.gov/oha/PH/PROVIDERPARTNERRESOURCES/EVALUATIONRESEARCH/DEATHWITHDIGNITYACT/Documents/year25.pdf.

8. Washington State Department of Health, "Death with Dignity Data 2021," https://doh.wa.gov/sites/default/files/2022-11/422-109-DeathWithDignityAct2021.pdf?uid=65223d84338b4.

9. Health Canada, *Third Annual Report on Medical Assistance in Dying in Canada 2021* (Ottawa: Government of Canada, 2022), https://www.canada.ca/en/health-canada/services/publications/health-system-services/annual-report-medical-assistance-dying-2021.html.

10. See, for example, Pereira, "Legalizing Euthanasia or Assisted Suicide," 38–45. Others suggest that such concerns, to date, have not been justified by the data we have. See Battin et al., "Legal Physician-Assisted Dying in Oregon and the Netherlands" and Norwood, Kisma, and Battin, "Vulnerability and the 'Slippery Slope' at the End-of-Life." I must admit that my review of the literature leaves me inconclusive about the current prevalence of abuse. It seems, on the whole, those who have had recourse to PAS or euthanasia tend to be well-educated, well-insured white men (see, e.g., the case of Dr. Wesley in chapter 1), who have typically actively participated in the process of securing access to life-ending prescriptions. Nevertheless, although I do not wish to make any strong arguments from silence, it is (a) unclear how the data might account for or fail to account for more ambiguous cases and (b) unclear that the practice has become widespread enough to affect cultural norms in the ways that PAS skeptics worry about. It is unlikely that our end-of-life practices, even if they incorporate PAS or euthanasia, will resemble Huxley's *Brave New World*, but it is also possible that the pressures that attend vulnerable populations are far subtler and more difficult to measure than we might suppose. This seems to be part of what is occurring in the Canadian context, with recent attempts to broaden access to medical assistance in dying (MAID) to nonterminal patients. See Raikin, "No Other Options."

11. See Sulmasy, "Transcript of IQ2 Debate."

12. Burns, "With Help, Conductor and Wife Ended Lives."

13. For a critique of the Groningen Protocol, see Jotkowitz and Glick, "The Groningen Protocol." For a more sympathetic perspective, see Lindemann and Verkerk, "Ending the Life of a Newborn."

14. For an example of this line of reasoning (which, however, does not address implications for PAS), see Hawkins and Emanuel, "Clarifying Confusions about Coercion."

15. Velleman, "Against the Right to Die." For another argument for this conclusion, see Schwartz, *The Paradox of Choice*.

16. Velleman, "Against the Right to Die," 672.

17. Velleman, "Against the Right to Die," 672.

18. Velleman, "Against the Right to Die," 672; emphasis original.

19. Velleman, "Against the Right to Die," 671–72; emphasis original.

20. Banner, *The Ethics of Everyday Life*, 116; emphasis original. James Mumford perceptively notes how the prevalence of the language of "choice" in debates about PAS undermines liberal commitments to the value of "inclusivity," especially when the perspective of the profoundly disabled is taken. See Mumford, *Vexed*. See also Moyse, *Resourcing Hope*.

21. Cited in Swinton, *Dementia*.

22. Callahan, *The Troubled Dream of Life*, 33–34.

23. See National Hospice and Palliative Care Organization (NHPCO), *Facts and Figures: Hospice in America, 2015 Edition* (Alexandria, VA: NHPCO, 2015). According to the report, "Length of service can be reported as both an average and a median. The median, however, is considered a more meaningful measure for understanding the experience of the typical patient since it is not influenced by outliers (extreme values)."

24. Taylor, *Sources of the Self*, 8.

25. See Taylor, *Modern Social Imaginaries*, 23. Compare Taylor, *A Secular Age*, chap. 4.

26. Taylor, *Sources of the Self*, ix.

27. Taylor, *Sources of the Self*, 121.

28. Taylor, *Sources of the Self*, 131. We should note that this is a highly contested reading of Augustine. For important critiques of Taylor on this point, see, for example, Hanby, *Augustine and Modernity*; Milbank, "Sacred Triads"; Mathewes, "Augustinian Anthropology."

29. Augustine, *De vera religione* XXXIX.72; emphasis added.

30. Taylor, *Sources of the Self*, 132; emphasis added.

31. Taylor, *Sources of the Self*, 171. Importantly, Locke makes *self-consciousness* the primary component of what it means to be a human person. Locke "refuses to identify the self or person with any substance, material or immaterial, but makes it depend on consciousness. . . . 'For it is by the consciousness it has of its present thoughts and action, that it is a *self* to *itself* now, and so will be the same self, as far as the same consciousness can extend to actions past and to come'" (172).

The centrality of self-consciousness to our modern notions of personhood are hard to overstate.

32. Taylor, *Sources of the Self*, 181.
33. Taylor, *Sources of the Self*, 181.
34. Taylor, *Sources of the Self*, 374.
35. Wordsworth, *The Prelude*.
36. Taylor, *Sources of the Self*, 384.
37. Such a claim immediately calls for nuance. For example, although the monks aspired to a form of spiritual and moral life that was generally not considered to be required of all baptized Christians (especially insofar as they aimed at a life of prayer and the attainment of the evangelical counsels of perfection, including poverty, chastity, and obedience), we must acknowledge that many monastic communities were equally dedicated to the shared tasks of daily life, including manual labor. *Ora et labora* goes the ancient Benedictine saying, and none can doubt it who have read the reflections of Brother Lawrence. See Brother Lawrence, *The Practice of the Presence of God*.
38. We have already noted how the Cartesian turn toward "inwardness" has important roots in Augustine's conviction that the best way to the God who infinitely surpasses me is to look within to the soul that bears God's image. Correlatively, the mechanistic view of the universe which culminated in Deism is importantly related to the theological voluntarism of Duns Scotus and the medieval nominalists. This deep history is important for understanding the nature of the concepts that seem to us to be common sense but for which we have a difficult time accounting. The theological sources may be lost to us in important ways. This is true of many aspects of the modern identity. According to Taylor, "In each case, the stimulus existed within Christian culture itself to generate these views which stand on the threshold. Augustinian inwardness stands behind the Cartesian turn, and the mechanistic universe was originally a demand of theology. The disengaged subject stands in a place already hollowed out for God; he takes a stance to the world which befits an image of the Deity. The belief in interlocking nature follows the affirmation of ordinary life, a central Judeo-Christian idea, and extends the centrally Christian notion that God's goodness consists in his stopping to seek the benefit of humans. What arises in each case is a conception which stands ready for a mutation, which will carry it outside the Christian faith altogether." See Taylor, *Sources of the Self*, 315.
39. Weber, *The Protestant Ethic and the Spirit of Capitalism*.
40. Taylor, *Sources of the Self*, 232.
41. Taylor, *Sources of the Self*, 394.
42. Kaufman, *Ordinary Medicine*, 7. To avoid confusion, it should be noted that the term "ethically necessary" is not being used as a precise category, arising from rigorous ethical analysis, as is the distinction between "optional" and "obliga-

tory" treatments in Beauchamp and Childress's *Principles of Biomedical Ethics*. Trained ethicists will be more careful and precise with the term than Kaufman is here. By "ethically necessary" she means that patients come to expect their use and physicians are unlikely to hesitate to provide such treatments.

43. Kaufman, *Ordinary Medicine*, 101; emphasis added.

44. Studies indicate that among those who request PAS, only about 22 percent cite the fear of pain as a motivating factor; nearly all of them cite fear of loss of control and autonomy. See Emanuel, "Four Myths about Doctor-Assisted Suicide."

45. For example, like many in the early church, we might simultaneously hold that the human being as "rational animal" garners a certain sort of respect not afforded to nonrational animals, while still subordinating this sort of dignity with a deeper dignity grounded extrinsically by the singular relationship that the human beings have with God—namely, that they are "chosen in Christ before the foundation of the world" (Eph 1:4).

46. Kenneth G. MacKendrick subjects this practice to critical scrutiny, arguing against the notions of individualism implicit in personal narratives. See MacKendrick, "Intersubjectivity and the Revival of Death."

47. Walter, "Facing Death without Tradition."

48. Banner, *The Ethics of Everyday Life*, 115.

49. Banner, *The Ethics of Everyday Life*, 115.

THREE. Persons, Freedom, and a Catholic Spirituality of Martyrdom

1. Battin, *Ending Life*, 6.

2. Initially promulgated by Pope John Paul II in 1996, it "aims at presenting an organic synthesis of the essential and fundamental contents of Catholic doctrine, as regards both faith and morals, in the light of the Second Vatican Council and the whole of the Church's Tradition. Its principal sources are the Sacred Scriptures, the Fathers of the Church, the liturgy, and the Church's Magisterium" (CCC, Prologue.3.11). *Catechism of the Catholic Church*.

3. Aquinas, *Summa theologica* IIa. IIae. Q.164, A.1.

4. Although Thomas thinks that the soul can achieve Beatitude (the *visio Dei*) apart from the body, he also holds that separated from the body, the soul is not yet perfected. "The desire of the separated soul is entirely at rest, as regards what is desired; since, to wit, it has that which satisfies its appetite. But it is not wholly at rest as regards the desirer, since it does not possess that good in every way that it would wish to possess it. Consequently, after the body has been resumed, happiness increases not in intensity but in extent" (Aquinas, *Summa theologica* Ia. IIae. Q.4, A.5).

5. See, for example, John Paul II, *Evangelium Vitae*, n47.
6. Compare United States Conference of Catholic Bishops, *Ethical and Religious Directives*, 29.
7. The *Declaration on Euthanasia* asserts that taking one's life is "equally as wrong as murder," though circumstantially, guilt for the act might be diminished, or even "completely remove[d]."
8. Compare John Paul II, *Evangelium Vitae*, 65.
9. In the fourth edition to the *Ethical and Religious Directives for Catholic Health Care Services*, issued in 2001, the U.S. Conference of Catholic Bishops noted that the withdrawal of AN&H from comatose or persistent vegetative state patients had not been settled by the magisterium. According to the *Directives* (2001), "hydration and nutrition are not morally obligatory either when they bring no comfort to a person who is imminently dying or when they cannot be assimilated by a person's body." This, however, had apparently changed by the time the fifth edition was published in 2009. By that time, Pope John Paul II had declared that to withhold AN&H from the patient in a permanent vegetative state is "true and proper euthanasia by omission" because it is known that death by starvation and dehydration is the only possible outcome. It is not possible in such a situation to regard the death that occurs as a foreseen but unintended consequence of the act of withdrawing AN&H. See John Paul II, *Address to the Participants*.

It should be noted that although this interpretation is widely considered to be the correct one, some have argued that it hinges on a misunderstanding of what Pope John Paul II was actually discussing in this particular address. For example, James T. Bretzke, S.J., argues that one must bear in mind a series of general guidelines for the "exegesis" of magisterial teachings. Following the Vatican II document *Lumen Gentium (The Dogmatic Constitution of the Church)*, he asserts that "the character of the teaching itself, the frequency with which the teaching is reaffirmed, and the manner in which the teaching is given" must each be considered in interpreting Church teaching. So, for example, a teaching frequently repeated over time may hold more authority than one that has only occasionally been articulated or that was once regularly taught but that over time has been increasingly ignored (e.g., the prohibition of interest as usurious). Likewise, an official dogma promulgated by a Church council or by the pope, speaking ex cathedra, carries much greater weight than, say, an informal address from the pope to a group of Italian midwives. Bretzke argues, in short, that the March 2004 address (and, in particular, the statement made there that AN&H "should be considered, in principle, ordinary and proportionate, and as such morally obligatory, insofar as and until it is seen to have attained its proper finality, which in the present case consists in providing nourishment to the patient and alleviation of suffering") must be read in light of other, more authoritative, explanations of "ordinary" and "extraordinary" treatments in, for example, the CDF's "*Iura et Bona*: Declaration on Euthanasia," John Paul II's *Evangelium Vitae*, and the *Catechism of the Catholic Church* (192). Bretzke concludes that "the main thrust of the address is not aimed at reversing the centuries-old tradition of ordinary and extraordinary means, which would have to be the case if in fact the pope meant that AN&H would have to be always administered regardless of the necessary subjective considerations of the individual patient's own benefit and burden calculus" (194). See Bretzke, "The Burden of Means." This conclusion is echoed by Cahill, "Catholicism, Death, and Modern Medicine."

10. Congregation for the Doctrine of the Faith, "Instruction on Respect for Human Life in Its Origin and on the Dignity of Procreation," February 22, 1987, https://www.academyforlife.va/content/dam/pav/documents/papi/documentisantasede/ENGLISH/donum_vitae_ENG.pdf.

11. Mauceri, "Euthanasia," 377.

12. This focus on the act is, in part, a reflection of the neoscholastic methodology that lies behind the magisterial teachings. As one commentator notes, the neoscholastic "manualist" tradition was "rooted, with some notable exceptions, not in the virtues or Sacred Scripture . . . but in the categories of law and moral obligation, which, in turn, contributed to legalism, moral minimalism, [and] a separation of moral theology from spirituality" (Latkovic, "Moral Theology," 716).

13. This is not to suggest that motive is irrelevant for morality. In addition to the "moral object," Roman Catholic moral theology considers the agent's motivation and the circumstances (including the consequences) of the act. An act that is morally neutral in its object but is performed with an evil intention is considered sinful, just as an act that is intrinsically evil in its moral object cannot be made legitimate by virtue of being performed with good intentions. See *Catechism of the Catholic Church*, 3.1.1.4.

14. See Pope John Paul II, *Veritatis Splendor*, chap. 4, pt. 2. See also May, *An Introduction to Moral Theology*, chap. 4. Compare Aquinas, *Summa theologiae*, 1–2, 18, 6.

15. For an elaboration of this argument, see Meilaender, "Euthanasia & Christian Vision."

16. John Paul II, *Evangelium Vitae*.

17. "The use of palliative care, including painkillers and sedatives, even if such use may shorten life, is morally licit" (John Paul II, *Evangelium Vitae*, 65).

18. See, for example, Beauchamp and Childress, *Principles of Biomedical Ethics*.

19. Congregation on the Doctrine of the Faith, *Declaration on Euthanasia*.

20. United States Conference of Catholic Bishops, *Ethical and Religious Directives*, 31.

21. Congregation on the Doctrine of the Faith, *Declaration on Euthanasia*.

22. Originally published in 1974, it was later included in a collection of essays. See McCormick, "To Save or Let Die," 341.

23. McCormick, "To Save or Let Die," 344–45.

24. McCormick, "To Save or Let Die," 345. The suggestion that a "quality of life" judgment is not only inevitable but also morally appropriate has invited criticism from other Roman Catholic moral theologians. Some have suggested that the introduction of quality-of-life judgments is dangerous insofar as it may slide from a judgment regarding the relative benefit of certain treatments for the patient to the relative worth of a person's life—a shift in focus that threatens to undermine the dignity of the human person and to endanger vulnerable populations. (See, e.g., Ramsey, *Ethics at the Edges of Life*, 172. Ramsey, though not himself a Roman Catholic moral theologian, represents a broader concern voiced by others.) Others suggest that life, as a basic good, always has value for a person, though it need not always be indefinitely prolonged. Although McCormick is aware of such arguments, he nevertheless argues that quality-of-life judgments are important and necessary (see McCormick, "The Quality of Life, the Sanctity of Life"). Indeed, he notes that the classification of a proposed treatment as "ordinary" or "extraordinary" in fact often hinges on a previous judgment about the kind of life the patient might expect to enjoy as a result of the treatment's implementation.

25. McCormick, "To Save or Let Die," 344.

26. Pope Pius XII, *Acta Apostalicae Sedis*, 49 (1957), 1031–32; emphasis added.

27. McCormick, "To Save or Let Die," 345.

28. McCormick, "To Save or Let Die," 346.

29. McCormick, "To Save or Let Die," 349. At this point, a few points could be made regarding McCormick's seeming equation of "humanity" and "relational potential." It first glance, it may seem as if McCormick is here making relational potentiality into a qualifying characteristic of human personhood—a position that would be troublesome, for example, to those influenced by disability theorists. McCormick, however, is not saying that a life that fails to demonstrate relationality falls below the threshold of human personhood (in "Letter to the Editor" of the *Hastings Center Report*), McCormick excoriates Joseph Fletcher for "annexing" an earlier reflection on human relationality for precisely this purpose) but rather that this human person lacks the relational quality that would make this life meaningful for him or her.

Additionally, McCormick notes that relational potential can be limited by external factors like prejudice and discrimination: "Life's potentiality for other values is dependent on two factors: those external to the individual, and the very condition of the individual. The former we can and must change to maximize individual potential. That is what social justice is all about. The latter we sometimes cannot alter" (348).

Finally, McCormick acknowledges a number of important caveats regarding quality-of-life judgments that press in a protectionist direction. Among these are the following: (1) Relational potential exists along a spectrum, and the valuation of relational potential is a matter of clinical judgment. There are many gray areas between the clear cases of anencephaly (no) and Down syndrome (yes); (2) As a clinical judgment, we must be aware of the potential for mistakes and therefore, when possible, err on the side of preserving life; (3) Allowing a child to die does mean that "some lives are more valuable than others" or that this particular life is "not worth living." "This is not a question about the inherent value of the individual. It is a question about whether this worldly existence will offer such a valued individual any hope of sharing those values for which physical life is the fundamental condition"; (4) It is not inherently objectionable, and indeed appropriate, that these decisions are made by parents with physicians, but (5) they should be made with the child's welfare alone in mind.

30. Rourke, "Personalism." Compare Wojtyła, *Acting Person*; Modras, "Thomistic Personalism"; and Merkle, "Personalism."

31. McCormick, "The Consistent Ethic of Life," 212.

32. According to McCormick, this principle originally referred to the "moral legitimacy of removing or curtailing a function or an organ for the good of the whole person" (*Health and Medicine in the Catholic Tradition*, 15). Although the term was coined by Pope Pius XII in 1952, the principle itself was employed by Thomas Aquinas.

33. Cahill, "Richard A. McCormick's 'To Save or Let Die,'" 135.

34. McCormick, *Health and Medicine in the Catholic Tradition*, 19; emphasis original.

35. Tollefson, "The New Natural Law Theory," 6. See also Grisez, *The Way of the Lord Jesus, Volume 1* and Finnis, *Moral Absolutes*.

36. Childress, "Religious Viewpoints," 131.

37. Cahill, "Richard A. McCormick's 'To Save or Let Die,'" 141–42.

38. Cahill, "Richard A. McCormick's 'To Save or Let Die,'" 142–43.

39. See, for example, McCormick, "Notes on Moral Theology," especially 73, in which he describes "the *practical absoluteness* of the prohibition against directly causing death in all terminal situations" (emphasis original).

40. McCormick, "Notes on Moral Theology," 76.

41. McCormick, "Notes on Moral Theology," 67.

42. See, for example, Tully, *Refined Consequentialism*.

43. McCormick was most often content to leave explicitly Christian doctrines in the background, but at times his writing took on a more theologically inflected tone. Often, this occurred in the context of discussion on end-of-life issues. In an article on

the relationship between theology and bioethics, McCormick argues that one should not expect faith to supply direct answers to the problems of "quandary ethics" so typical of bioethical literature. Rather, faith informs ethics at a deeper level—at the level of a meaning-transforming story, providing "perspectives, themes, insights, not always or chiefly direct action guides." McCormick, "Theology and Bioethics," 7.

44. McCormick, "Theology and Bioethics," 9; emphasis added.

45. McCormick, "Theology and Bioethics," 9. Maura Ryan points to the way McCormick offers resources for a "spirituality of limits" that might be helpful for Christians thinking through issues of assisted reproduction and end-of-life ethics. See Ryan, *Ethics and Economics of Assisted Reproduction*, 165.

46. McCormick, "Physician-Assisted Suicide," 1132; emphasis original.

47. Rahner, *On the Theology of Death*. Hereafter cited in text. Rahner reflected on death and dying numerous times throughout his life, writing at least nine articles and one monograph on the subject between 1957 and 1976. These works are listed in Jones, *Approaching the End*, 149n8–9.

48. Here, Rahner's thought reflects a long line of existentialist-phenomenological reflection on the interplay between freedom and finitude, running from Kierkegaard and Heidegger through Reinhold Niebuhr and Paul Tillich. (See, e.g., Kierkegaard, *The Concept of Anxiety*; Kierkegaard, *The Sickness unto Death*; Heidegger, *Being and Time*; Heidegger, *The Fundamental Concepts of Metaphysics*; R. Niebuhr, *The Nature and Destiny of Man*; and Tillich, *Systematic Theology, Volume 2*.) It is no wonder that Peter C. Phan describes Rahner's theology of death during this period as "individualist-existentialist." See Phan, "Eschatology."

49. See Meilaender, *Should We Live Forever?*, chap. 1.

50. Craigo-Snell, *Silence, Love, and Death*, 25.

51. Mulhall, *Philosophical Myths of the Fall*, 50.

52. According to Heidegger, "the ending that we have in view when we speak of death, does not signify a being-at-the-end of Dasein, but rather a *being toward the end* [*Sein zum Ende*] of this being. Death is a way to be that Dasein takes over as soon as it is." *Being and Time*, 236.

53. Heidegger, *Being and Time*, 248.

54. Remenyi, "Death as the Limit to Life and Thought."

55. Craigo-Snell, *Silence, Love, and Death*, 126.

56. Ochs, "Death as Act."

57. In saying this, I recognize that there are forms of surrender that do not indicate trust but rather resignation or fear of brute force. This heteronomous surrender, however, is not what is displayed in Christ's crucifixion. Although the empire and the Pharisees thought Jesus's death was simply suffered, it is precisely the mystery of faith that Christ "gave himself for us to redeem us" (Titus 2:14).

58. Craigo-Snell, *Silence, Love, and Death*, 132; emphasis added.

59. Rahner elaborates the nature of freedom as "mysterious interplay between action and passion" in the following quotation: "The freedom which is exercised on the physical plane is, in fact, that freedom by which man lays himself open to intervention from without, submits to control by another power or powers. They [*sic*] physical side of man's nature constitutes the sphere in which the interplay takes place of action from within himself and passion as imposed from without. As a physical being endowed with freedom man has to take cognizance of the fact that he occupies an intermediary position. He is neither wholly self-directing nor wholly subject to control by another, but half-way between these two. The mysterious interplay between action and passion in the exercise of human freedom appears above all in the fact that it is precisely at the very point at which man freely achieves his own perfection that he is, at the same time, most wholly subject to control by another. The ultimate act of freedom, in which he decides his own fate totally and irrevocably, is the act in which he either willingly accepts or definitively rebels against his own utter impotence, in which he is utterly subject to the control of a mystery which cannot be expressed—that mystery which we call God. In death man is totally withdrawn from himself. Every power, down to the last vestige of a possibility, of autonomously controlling his own destiny is taken away from him. Thus the exercise of freedom taken as a whole is summed up at this point in one single decision: whether he yields everything up or whether everything is taken from him by force, whether he responds to this radical deprivation of all power by uttering his assent in faith and hope to the nameless mystery which we call God, or protests against this fall into helplessness, and, because of his disbelief, supposes that he is falling into the abyss of nothingness when in reality he is falling into the unfathomable depths of God." See Rahner, "On Christian Dying," 289–90.

60. Pinckaers suggests that moral theologians adopt a "broader conception of spirituality" than they typically have. By spirituality, Pinckaers means "the study of the Christian life and its development insofar as that life is placed under the direction of the Holy Spirit." See Pinckaers, *Spirituality of Martyrdom*, 13–14. Hereafter cited in text.

61. See, for example, Wicker, "Conflict and Martyrdom" and "The Drama of Martyrdom."

62. See, for example, Hovey, *To Share in the Body*.

63. Pinckaers, *Spirituality of Martyrdom*, 2, 11. Pinckaers draws this conclusion from an interpretation (originally put forward by Augustine) of the Beatitudes, which holds the eighth Beatitude ("Blessed are those who are persecuted for righteousness's sake, for theirs is the kingdom of Heaven") as the culmination and summation of the Beatitudes as a whole.

FOUR. Karl Barth on Agency in Dying: Accepting Creaturely Finitude

1. See McCormack, *Orthodox and Modern*, 11. See also Kapic and McCormack, *Mapping Modern Theology* and Sherman, *The Shift to Modernity*.
2. Schleiermacher had earlier declared his intention "to establish an eternal covenant between the living Christian faith and completely free, independent scientific inquiry, so that faith does not hinder science and science does not exclude faith." See Schleiermacher, *On the* Glaubenslehre, 64.
3. McCormack. *Orthodox and Modern*, 17; emphasis original.
4. Sonderegger, "Creation," 98.
5. Sonderegger, "Creation," 100.
6. Sonderegger, "Creation," 100. In recent years, academic theology has seen a marked uptick in interest in the doctrine of creation and in its implications for an understanding of human beings *as creatures*. This renewed attention to the doctrine of creation has multiple sources and manifestations. Some of these works are motivated by an increasing ecological consciousness, which attempts to correct for a perceived overly anthropocentric doctrine of creation in the tradition (see, e.g., Clough, *On Animals*; and Bauckham, *Living with Other Creatures*). Some are written from a related concern to incorporate the latest insights of evolutionary science into theological anthropology (see, e.g., Deane-Drummond, *Christ and Evolution*; Deane-Drummond and Clough, *Creaturely Theology*; and Moore, *Divinanimality*). Feminist theology and disability literature have also turned attention toward the importance of embodiment and vulnerability (see, e.g., Creamer, *Disability and Christian Theology*). Others are driven by dogmatic and exegetical concerns (see, e.g., Kelsey, *Eccentric Existenc*e; and Moltmann, *God in Creation*).
7. See Osborn, *Death before the Fall*.
8. This phrase was originally applied to Barth's theology by Fergus Kerr. See Kerr, *Immortal Longings*, 23–24.
9. Summing up the view of second-century church father Tatian, church historian Jaroslav Pelikan goes so far as to refer to "the gospel of death [that] announces to men the gracious message that they will die once and for all" and to claim "the message of the church to the Greek world, then, is: Accept the arc of existence and be conformed to the shape of death!" See Pelikan, *The Shape of Death*, 20, 25.
10. See, for example, Berkouwer, *The Triumph of Grace*, 155.
11. This quotation is from the editors' preface to *CD* III.2. The editors continue, "Whatever else may be said about creation rests on what is said explicitly about the relationship of God and man. . . . Only from this standpoint can theology speak of the rest of creation" (*CD* III.2, vii). In his own preface to the same volume, Barth claims he recognizes the radical nature of his Christological under-

standing of creation and the creature, which "deviates even more widely from dogmatic tradition than in the doctrine of predestination in [*CD* II.2]. None of the older or more recent fathers known to me was ready to take the way to a *theological knowledge* of man which I regard as the only possible one" (*CD* III.2, ix; emphasis added). Compare Tanner, "Creation and Providence."

12. Genesis 1 also describes creation in terms of God setting a definite limit to the "chaos." Barth affirms, in principle, the doctrine of creation ex nihilo and the resulting implication that all that has been created by God is good and ordered toward God's good purposes (*CD* III.1, 99–100). He rejects the idea that God first created "chaos," only to later shape it into orderly creation. The "formless and void" (Gen 1:2) "can have reality only as that which by God's decision and operation has been rejected and has disappeared" (*CD* III.1, 102). "Chaos," insofar as it exists, does so only as a "possibility negated and rejected by God" (*CD* III.1, 109). Discussing Genesis 1:3–5, Barth notes something puzzling in the text—namely, that God both creates and names "light," but God only names "darkness" (i.e., "night"). Nowhere does it say that God *created* darkness. This does not mean that the darkness presents a formidable challenge to the light or to the God who created light. No, the God who is "the Creator of light is also the Lord of darkness. The fact that darkness, and the chaos which it represents, is not His creation does not mean that it has escaped or evaded Him" (*CD* III.1, 126).

13. Barth had a marked preference for temporal and historical language over against the more "substantialist" language typical of Greek metaphysical thought. As Eberhard Busch explains, for Barth, God "*is*," but "his being is not a special case within a general concept of being.... Nor is his being static, so that his activity would be something external and over against him, which he could do without" (*The Great Passion*, 47). Thus, Barth's "actualism" refers to his refusal to consider essence (whether divine or human) apart from act. Further, for Barth, the fundamental act that forms the ontic basis for all we can know about God is God's covenantal relationship with humanity, which occurs in the person (i.e., history) of Jesus Christ. Therefore, not only God and humankind but also their relationship must be described in actualistic terms. In the words of George Hunsinger, "Negatively [actualism] means that we human beings have no ahistorical relationship to God, and that we also have no capacity in and of ourselves to enter into fellowship with God. An ahistorical relationship would be a denial of God's activity, and an innate capacity for fellowship would be a denial of God's sovereignty. Positively, therefore, our relationship with God must be understood in active, historical terms, and it must be a relationship given to us strictly from the outside.... Our relationship to God is therefore an event" (*How to Read Karl Barth*, 31). The issue of the possible implications of Barth's actualism for his understanding of divine ontology (i.e., the being of God) is a matter of considerable

and vigorous debate in Barth studies. See, for example, McCormack, *Orthodox and Modern* and Hunsinger, *Reading Barth with Charity.*

14. See Mangina, *Karl Barth*, 71; and Van Driel, *Incarnation Anyway*, especially 63–117. Compare *CD* II.2, 133–45.

15. Barth once claimed that upon arriving in heaven, he would seek out the great theological saints (Augustine, Aquinas, Calvin) only after sitting at Mozart's feet. "It may be," he wrote, "that when the angels go about their task of praising God, they play only Bach. I am sure, however, that when they are together *en famille*, they play Mozart and that then too our dear Lord listens with special pleasure." See Barth, *Wolfgang Amadeus Mozart*. It is also said that late in life, Barth experienced a mystical vision of Mozart gazing at him during a performance.

16. Barth, *Wolfgang Amadeus Mozart*, 33.

17. Barth, *Wolfgang Amadeus Mozart*, 55–56.

18. Barth, *Wolfgang Amadeus Mozart*, 57.

19. On Barth's account of evil as "nothingness," see Burnett, *The Westminster Handbook to Karl Barth*, 68–69; McDowell, "Much Ado about Nothing"; Reuther, "The Left Hand of God"; and Wolterstorff, "Barth on Evil."

20. Kaltwasser, "The Measure of Our Days."

21. Barth, *The Epistle to the Romans*. Hereafter cited in text as *Romans* II.

22. This comment, attributed to Roman Catholic theologian Karl Adam, was made in reference to the first edition but, needless to say, applies equally well to the more widely read second edition.

23. See Barth's essay "Evangelical Theology in the Nineteenth Century," in *The Humanity of God*, 14. On Barth's general sense of "alienation" from liberal theology during this period, see McCormack, *Karl Barth's Critically Realistic Dialectical Theology*, 78–125.

24. Letter from Karl Barth to Wilhelm Herrmann, November 4, 1914, cited in McCormack, *Karl Barth's Critically Realistic Dialectical Theology*, 113.

25. McCormack, *Karl Barth's Critically Realistic Dialectical Theology*, 113.

26. McCormack, *Karl Barth's Critically Realistic Dialectical Theology*, 246.

27. Barth employs the Kantian noumena-phenomena distinction to preserve the divine prerogative in the event of revelation. In Kantian terms, God must become "intuitable as the Unintuitable." In Barth's own day, the radical emphasis on *diastasis* and *Krisis* invited the charge of theological skepticism. Many wondered whether the theology of *Romans* II rendered God completely unknowable. Although understandable, this charge misses the point. For Barth stresses repeatedly that although we cannot cross the line of death to get to God, God has already crossed it to get to us. Revelation occurs! On Kant's influence on Barth, see McCormack, *Karl Barth's Critically Realistic Dialectical Theology*, 245.

28. One potentially fruitful way of framing this aspect of Barth's thought is to see *Romans* II as a radicalization of Luther's *theologia crucis*. Because our fundamental sin is the denial of the limits of human possibility, we must be dashed against these limits to be shown that God's faithfulness extends to the exact place where we would least expect it.

29. A similar point was made by Saint Irenaeus, *Against Heresies*, III.xxiii.6.

30. There are a number of useful monographs and general introductions to Barth's ethical theory. See, for example, Biggar, *The Hastening that Waits*; Clough, *Ethics in Crisis*; Werpehowski, *Karl Barth and Christian Ethics*; Haddorff, *Christian Ethics as Witness*; Migliore, *Commanding Grace*; Webster, *Barth's Moral Theology*; Nimmo, *Being in Action*; and McKenny, *The Analogy of Grace*. For a more critical engagement, see Rose, *Ethics with Barth*.

31. See Puffer, "Taking Exception."

32. This claim rests on an interpretation of Barth's use of the term *Grenzfall* (i.e., "limit situation") that is occluded by certain editorial and translation choices in the original English translation of *CD* III.4. According to John Hare, Barth draws "the distinction between boundary case (*Grenzfall*) and exception (*Ausnahme*), and then he [denies] that the boundary case is an exception. Unfortunately, this is disguised in the English translation, which translates *Grenzfall* as 'exception.' Barth goes to great length to interpret what look like exceptions (in the cases of abortion, tyrannicide, self-defense, and war) as actually strange or paradoxical instances of the command to protect life" (*God's Command*, 152n31). Compare Puffer, "Taking Exception."

33. Ridenour, "The Coming of Age," 160.

34. Ridenour, "The Coming of Age," 160.

35. Ridenour, "The Coming of Age," 161.

36. See Vanstone, *The Stature of Waiting*, chap. 6, "The God Who Waits."

37. Ridenour, "The Coming of Age," 164.

FIVE. Stanley Hauerwas on Agency in Dying: Ethics of Dispossession

1. Hauerwas and Burrell, "From System to Story," 20.

2. In addition to his early Gifford Lectures (*With the Grain of the Universe*), Hauerwas also describes his appreciation for Karl Barth at length in what is at the time of this writing his most recent (and possibly final) book, *Fully Alive*.

3. The significance of the essay should not be missed. The essay form reflects Hauerwas's conviction that the human being exists as a contingent, time-bound, and finite creature. As Adam Joyce points out, in his preference for essay over system,

"Hauerwas doesn't create a universe of discourse but instead shows one essay at a time how we can go on speaking as Christians as certain forms of Christendom die. . . . Ultimately, it is the story of Christ that guides the Christian pilgrim in the act of 'going on.' This story is what provides the church with the direction, the sense of where we are walking to and why we are walking. Yet we need more than a story. We don't just tell the story—we must reflect on it—and the essay is a genre especially fit for reflecting on the story and assisting with the act of going on. It is a form of speech, a mode of theology, appropriate for the Christian sojourner, the pilgrim" ("You Always Begin an Essay"). For more on Hauerwas's use of the essay form, see Hauerwas, *Truthfulness and Tragedy*, 3 and Hauerwas, *Sanctify Them in the Truth*, 9. Compare also Hauerwas, *The Work of Theology*, 23–24.

4. Hauerwas, *Truthfulness and Tragedy*, 8.

5. Hauerwas, *Truthfulness and Tragedy*, 9. Hauerwas drives home his critique of the "standard account of moral rationality" in the essay, cowritten with David Burrell, "From System to Story," 15–39.

6. See Stout, *Ethics after Babel*, 5–6, 60–81.

7. Hauerwas, *The Peaceable Kingdom*, 17, 1.

8. Barth, *Church Dogmatics*, II.2, 518.

9. Gustafson, *An Examined Faith*, 64.

10. Hauerwas, *The Peaceable Kingdom*, 116.

11. Hauerwas, *Truthfulness and Tragedy*, 170.

12. Hauerwas, *Vision and Virtue*, 2.

13. Hauerwas, *Truthfulness and Tragedy*, 177. In statements such as these, of course, Hauerwas overstates his case. In actual fact, parents and physicians alike are typically willing and able to recognize and tolerate a wide range of potential outcomes short of withdrawing treatment. We may qualify Hauerwas's point by claiming that it stands to the degree that people hold to such "Promethean" assumptions about parenting. It seems even if many people uncritically uphold such a view of parenting, these assumptions are often challenged by the experience of bearing a critically ill child.

14. Hauerwas, *Truthfulness and Tragedy*, 178.

15. Hauerwas and Bondi, "Memory, Community, and the Reasons for Living," 579, 582.

16. The language of "grammar" reveals the profound influence of Wittgenstein on Hauerwas. See Kallenberg, *Ethics as Grammar*. Compare Hauerwas, *The Peaceable Kingdom*, xxi and Hauerwas, *Wilderness Wanderings*, 145.

17. Hauerwas and Bondi, "Memory, Community, and the Reasons for Living," 582.

18. Hauerwas and Bondi, "Memory, Community, and the Reasons for Living," 587.

19. Namely, in our time, "the voluntary taking of one's own life has itself become a way of life in order to let people play out false stories of bravery and heroism, to sustain [a] hollow sense of sacrifice. . . . There is nothing wrong with being a burden!" Hauerwas and Bondi, "Memory, Community, and the Reasons for Living," 593.

20. Hauerwas and Bondi, "Memory, Community, and the Reasons for Living," 596–97.

21. Hauerwas, *Dispatches from the Front*, 6. Compare Hauerwas, "Situation Ethics, Moral Notions, and Moral Authority."

22. Hauerwas, *Truthfulness and Tragedy*, 10.

23. Hauerwas, *The Peaceable Kingdom*, 16, 149.

24. Nakashima, *The Soul of a Tree*, xxi.

25. Matthew B. Crawford has drawn attention to the ways in which such craftsmanship relies on the existence of communities of skilled practice, where "competence rests on an apprehension of real features of the world, as refracted through some set of human needs/desires and corresponding technologies." To be formed within such craft traditions, argues Crawford, is to become oriented toward the material world in a way that contrasts with the dominant forms of modern epistemology. See Crawford, *The World beyond Your Head*, 209. Compare Crawford, *Shop Class as Soulcraft*.

26. Hauerwas, *The Peaceable Kingdom*, 29–30.

27. Hauerwas, *The Peaceable Kingdom*, 99, 100. It is interesting to note that in the course of explaining the methodological connection between truthfulness and community, Hauerwas explicitly discusses suicide and euthanasia. He notes the central importance in our own time of keeping alive "the language of gift of life," which "liberal society has little consistent reason to continue." If, in fact, liberal society continues to hold a negative view toward self-killing, it does so on the (false) presumption that "survival is a central virtue of individual and social existence." The church, "by striving to remain a community were [sic] 'suicide' can be used in a morally accurate manner, thus hold out an alternative to wider society" (*Truthfulness and Tragedy*, 10–11).

28. Hauerwas, *Truthfulness and Tragedy*, 10.

29. Hauerwas, "Can Democracy Be Christian?"

30. See Hauerwas, "Politics, Vision, and the Common Good" and "Theology and the New American Culture," in *Vision and Virtue*, as well as "The Church and Liberal Democracy," in *A Community of Character*.

31. Hauerwas, "Democratic Time," 538. This is not to say that Christians should be wholly uninterested in making critical distinctions between various forms of polity and in matters of public policy. Although Christians, if they are faithful (according to Hauerwas), must be committed to nonviolence, they may also recognize that the sphere of governmental authority goes beyond simply wielding the sword. For this reason, Christians "can ask that those in power be just, care for the orphans and widows, and use the least violent means possible to secure order" (540). In this way, they can not only witness to the state but also "participate" in government (540).

32. Hauerwas, *Truthfulness and Tragedy*, 10.
33. Hauerwas, *Dispatches from the Front*, 166–67.
34. Hauerwas, *Truthfulness and Tragedy*, 12.
35. See Hauerwas, "Medicine as a Tragic Profession," in *Truthfulness and Tragedy*.
36. See Bishop, "Finitude."
37. Hauerwas, *Truthfulness and Tragedy*, 190.
38. Hauerwas, "Preaching as though We Had Enemies," 48.
39. Compare Rawls, *A Theory of Justice*. Hauerwas notes that "the story that we have no story except the story we chose when we thought we had no story" is "inspired by Rawls's account of the original position." See Hauerwas, "Hauerwas on 'Hauerwas and the Law,'" 250.
40. Michael J. Sandel, "The Procedural Republic and the Unencumbered Self."
41. Carter, "Must Liberalism Be Violent?," 201.
42. Hauerwas, "Hauerwas on 'Hauerwas and the Law,'" 241.
43. Hauerwas, *Truthfulness and Tragedy*, 200.
44. Hauerwas and Pinches, "Practicing Patience," 353.
45. Hauerwas, *Suffering Presence*, 78.
46. Hauerwas and Pinches, "Practicing Patience," 354.
47. Hauerwas, *Naming the Silences*, 98–99.
48. Hauerwas, *Suffering Presence*, 68.
49. Hauerwas, "Finite Care," 331.
50. Hauerwas, *Naming the Silences*, 62. This is what Hauerwas means when, in another place, he writes that "*modern* medicine was formed by a modern culture that forced upon medicine the impossible role of bandaging the wounds of societies that are built upon the premise that God does not matter." See Hauerwas and Pinches, "Practicing Patience," 352; emphasis original. Hauerwas's account of "anthropodicy" is heavily indebted to Becker's *The Structure of Evil*.
51. Hauerwas, *Truthfulness and Tragedy*, 182.
52. Hauerwas, *Naming the Silences*, 64.
53. Quoted in Hauerwas, *Dispatches from the Front*, 165–66.

Notes to Pages 101–105   173

54. As Hauerwas notes, "The philosophical name we give to this compassion as an ethical alternative is sometimes called utilitarianism." It is instructive, in this regard, to consider Peter Singer's controversial defense of infanticide. It is from Singer's utilitarian ethics that we get one of the strongest arguments in favor of infanticide and, especially, of terminating the life of disabled newborn infants in cases when birth abnormalities "turn the normally joyful event of birth into a threat to the happiness of the parents, and any other children they may have" (*Practical Ethics*, 183). According to Singer, because such infants lack rationality, autonomy, and self-consciousness, it is permissible to consider other factors in one's moral evaluation of infanticide. If, then, from the perspective of the parents, the death of the child would be more a cause of relief than grief, then this may be counted as a reason for the acceptability of ending the child's life (183).

55. Hauerwas, *Dispatches from the Front*, 165.
56. Hauerwas, *Dispatches from the Front*, 165.
57. Hauerwas, *The Peaceable Kingdom*, 120.
58. Hauerwas, *The Peaceable Kingdom*, 120. This "casuistry" helps explain the importance in the Christian tradition of the lives of the saints. For this process "requires the imaginative testing of our habits of life against the well-lived and virtuous lives of others. It is from such testing that we learn what kinds of situations we may well have to anticipate as entailed by the narrative and community of which we are a part. Attending to such lives does not mean that we try to imitate others, though certainly imitation may be useful, but by letting those lives form our own we learn what our particular way of embodying the story entails. . . . We must let their lives imaginatively challenge our own" (121).
59. Hauerwas, *Vision and Virtue*, 167.
60. Hauerwas, *Vision and Virtue*, 177.
61. Hauerwas, *Vision and Virtue*, 178.
62. Hauerwas, "Religious Concepts," 332.
63. On Hauerwas's understanding of "witness," see Hauerwas and Pinches, "Witness."
64. Hauerwas, "Religions Concepts," 332.
65. Hauerwas and Bondi, "Memory, Community, and Reasons for Living," 588.
66. Hauerwas, "Finite Care," 332.
67. Hauerwas, *Vision and Virtue*, 183.
68. Hays, Foreword.
69. On the centrality of the chapter, see Hauerwas's introductory remarks: "Everything I have done in this book has been preparation for this chapter. . . . [All that precedes] have been attempts to establish a framework that can help us understand the moral significance of Jesus' life, death, and resurrection" (*Peaceable*

Kingdom, 72). On the centrality of the book, see Cartwright, "Afterword," 627; Dean, *For the Life of the World*, 50n204; and Hauerwas, *Peaceable Kingdom*, xvi (hereafter cited in text in this section).

70. Even more, Hauerwas argues, the cry of dereliction in particular reveals the nature of the kingdom. According to Hauerwas, "these words from the cross, and the cross itself, mean that the Father is to be found when all traces of power, at least as we understand power, are absent; that the Spirit's authoritative witness is *most clearly revealed* when all forms of human authority are lost; and that God's power and authority is to be found exemplified in this captive under the sentence of death." See Hauerwas, *Cross Shattered Christ*, 64; emphasis original. Dean rightly highlights the deeply Lutheran overtones of *theologia crucis* in this passage. See Dean, *For the Life of the World*, 62.

71. Hauerwas, *The Peaceable Kingdom*, 87; emphasis added. For Hauerwas, salvation is effected precisely through this particular act of dispossession. On this point, Hauerwas is particularly influenced by John Howard Yoder. Drawing on the work of Hendrikus Berkhof, Yoder explains the significance of the cross in the following way: "On the cross [Jesus] 'disarmed' the Powers, 'made a public example of them and thereby triumphed over them.'. . . It is precisely in the crucifixion that the true nature of the Powers has come to light. Previously they were accepted as the most basic and ultimate realities, as the gods of the world. Never had it been perceived, nor could it have been perceived, that this belief was founded on deception. . . . Now they are unmasked as false gods by their encounter with Very god; they are made a public spectacle. Thus Christ has 'triumphed over them.' The unmasking is actually already their defeat. . . . The concrete evidence of this triumph is that at the cross Christ has 'disarmed' the Powers. The weapon from which they heretofore derived their strength is struck out of their hands. This weapon was the power of illusion, their ability to convince us that they were the divine regents of the world, ultimate certainty and ultimate direction, ultimate happiness and the ultimate duty for small, dependent humanity. Since Christ we know that this is illusion." See Yoder, *The Politics of Jesus*, 146–47. Quoted in N. Kerr, *Christ, History and Apocalyptic*, 142.

72. This phrase invokes the famous interchange between H. Richard Niebuhr and his brother Reinhold Niebuhr on whether "doing nothing" could be a theologically meaningful response to the Japanese invasion of Manchuria. See H. Niebuhr, "The Grace of Doing Nothing," and R. Niebuhr, "Must We Do Nothing?"

73. To forestall one obvious objection, a further point about the idea of dispossession is in order. It might be claimed that to reduce Christian discipleship to an idea like "dispossession" makes the mistake of portraying the Christian life as overly ascetic, world denying, and grim. Perhaps there is something to this charge if

we allow that Hauerwas is guilty of such a wholesale "reduction." But one cannot deny that dispossession is a recurrent theme in Christian spirituality. "Taking up one's cross," "dying to self," "crucifying the flesh"—these all refer to a spiritual process of "mortification" that should not be ignored. Furthermore, Hauerwas provides a cogent argument that the particular form of dispossession he advocates is intrinsically related to our capacity for joy: "[For] nonviolence requires life-long training in being dispossessed of all that I think secures my significance and safety. And the irony is that the more we lose, the greater the possibility we have for living life joyfully. For joy is the disposition that comes from our readiness always to be surprised; or put even more strongly, joy is the disposition that comes from our realization that we can trust in surprises for the sustaining of our lives. Perhaps the most remarkable aspect of learning to live joyfully is that we learn to see the simple and most common aspects of our existence, such as our friends, our spouses, our children, as sheer gifts to which we have no right but who are nonetheless present to us. Thus just as surely as peaceableness is a training to be patient in the face of the tragic, it is also learning to live joyfully in the face of the tragic."
See, Hauerwas, *The Peaceable Kingdom*, 148.

74. Dispossession may have metaethical significance. It is instructive to consider the treatment of Hauerwas's "ethics" above in light of the idea of dispossession. When we do, it becomes clear that Hauerwas's postliberal, nonfoundationalist mode of reflection is an attempt to do ethics "out of control."

75. L'Arche (The Ark) is a network of homes where persons with disabilities (often severe cognitive disabilities) live in close proximity and intentional community with others who assist them. Of course, mention of L'Arche requires mention of L'Arche's founder, Jean Vanier, who, after his death, was revealed to have abused his power and authority and to have participated in sexual misconduct with multiple adult assistants and nuns over the course of his career. Vanier was not the first of Hauerwas's heroes whose history of abuse has been revealed. John Howard Yoder had a similar pattern of behavior. In light of these scandals, I have wrestled with whether to excise references to both figures from this book. In the end, I decided to keep them in. Especially with Vanier, I did not want to lose the good witness of the L'Arche communities themselves, which ought not to be tarnished in the aftermath of Vanier's behavior. For more on the problem with such "tainted legacies," see Guth, *The Ethics of Tainted Legacies*.

76. Cartwright, "Stanley Hauerwas's Essays," 633n12.

77. Hauerwas and Vanier, *Living Gently in a Violent World*.

78. Hauerwas, "What Love Looks Like." Compare Hauerwas, "Disability: An Attempt to Think With," in *Approaching the End*, 222–36 and Le Pichon, "The Sign of Contradiction," 96.

79. Hauerwas and Pinches, "Practicing Patience," 349. Hereafter cited in text in this section.

80. For an illuminating essay on this, see Wannenwetsch, "Loving the Limit."

81. Hauerwas and McKenney, "Doing Nothing Gallantly," in *Approaching the End*, 200–221.

82. Hauerwas and Pinches, "Memory, Community, and the Reasons for Living," 587–88.

83. Murdoch, *The Sovereignty of Good*, 36.

SIX. Prayer, Baptism, and Eucharist

1. The iconography of the ancient Church powerfully depicts the centrality of Christ's death in its depiction of the nativity. In many early nativity icons, Mary is seen stooping over the infant Jesus who is swaddled in a manger. The location, however, is not in a stable but in a cave. The manger looks suspiciously like a coffin and the swaddling clothes like grave clothes. The message is clear: Jesus came to die — in fact, his entire life and incarnation is in a sense his subjecting himself to human mortality and suffering. Thanks to Joe Lenow for this point.

2. C. S. Lewis, "Membership." For a similar articulation of this dynamic, see Williams, *Resurrection*.

3. Lysaught, "Suffering in Communion with Christ," 61.

4. Compare Lustig, "Prescribing Prayer?"

5. Lysaught, "Suffering in Communion with Christ," 71.

6. Coakley, "Prayer as Divine Propulsion," emphasis added. This section includes material from my article, "Gentle Space-Making."

7. Westphal, "Prayer as the Posture," 15. Theologian Alan Lewis echoes this thought in his reflection on the Lord's Prayer as a recognition of creaturely dependence: "Thus by the very act of prayer for daily bread the priestly, interceding church challenges modernity's myth of autonomy and self-sufficiency, our promethean belief in our own capacities to satisfy every need with our own resourcefulness and ingenuity, and secure the future for ourselves and our planetary home without a humble recognition of dependence, fragility, and accountability, or any expression of thanksgiving." A. Lewis, *Between Cross and Resurrection*, 399.

8. Kelsey, *Eccentric Existence*, 109.

9. *The Cloud of Unknowing*, 4. Hereafter cited in text.

10. Coakley, *Powers and Submissions*.

11. Coakley, *Powers and Submissions*, 45.

12. Coakley, *Powers and Submissions*, 34; emphasis original.

13. See Hampson, *Theology and Feminism*, 155.
14. Consider, for example, the poem "My First Name" by Susan Harlan:

> No, you can't call me
> By my first name,
> And yes,
> I know that
> A male professor
> Told you that titles
> Are silly
> Because a certain genre
> Of man
> Is always dying
> To performatively
> Divest himself
> Of his easily won
> Authority.

15. Coakley, *Powers and Submissions*, 35–36.
16. Coakley, *Powers and Submissions*, 4.
17. See Ward, "Suffering and Incarnation," 163–80. The double genitive is intentionally ambiguous.
18. Ward, "Suffering and Incarnation," 171.
19. Ward, "Suffering and Incarnation," 174.
20. See McCarty, "Diagnosis and Therapy."
21. Wasson et al., "Physician, Know Thyself," 83.
22. Wasson et al., "Physician, Know Thyself," 85.
23. Wasson et al., "Physician, Know Thyself," 83.
24. Wasson et al., "Physician, Know Thyself," 84.
25. Martin Luther, as quoted in Barth, *Epistle to the Romans*, 194.
26. Williams, *Tokens of Trust*, 112.
27. The following paragraphs are deeply indebted to Medley, "Always Carrying."
28. Williams, "The Nature of a Sacrament," in *On Christian Theology*, 204. Quoted in Medley, "Always Carrying," 477.
29. See Lysaught, "Witnessing Christ," 248. Quoted in Medley, "Always Carrying," 491.
30. Gregory, *Salvation at Stake*, 132. Quoted in Medley, "Always Carrying," 479. The martyr, Medley elaborates, demonstrates "'an *unwillingness* to grab hold of a hand on history and a *willingness* to accept the cost of this decision.' The logic of such a witness is 'the antithesis' of 'self-directed choice'" (479; emphasis original),

quoting both Toole, *Waiting for Godot in Sarajevo*, 215 and Huebner, *A Precarious Peace*, 139.

31. For a magisterial treatment on this theme, see Kelsey, *Eccentric Existence*.

32. Banner, "Scripts for Modern Dying," 252. Banner makes this particular point in a critical commentary on the movie *Still Alice*, but it applies to the language of "death before death" more generally as well. Compare Holton, "Memory, Persons, Dementia."

33. J. S. Taylor, "On Recognition, Caring and Dementia."

34. Personal hygiene and maintaining a clean appearance was a central part of my wife's grandfather's identity. When he was dying in hospice, her family accumulated a half dozen electric razors so that no matter where he found himself in his apartment, he would be able to find a way to shave. For more on the process of "upholding identity," see Lindemann, *Holding and Letting Go*.

35. Medley, "Always Carrying," 479.

36. N. Kerr, *Christ, History and Apocalyptic*, 195.

37. Banner, "Scripts for Modern Dying," 254.

38. Cavanaugh, "Killing for the Eucharist."

39. At his conversion, Augustine felt the Lord say to him, "I am the food of grown men; grow and you shall feed upon me; nor shall you change me, like the food of your flesh, into yourself, but you shall be changed into me." See Augustine, *Confessions*, VII.10.16.

40. Concannon, "Eschatological Implications," 888.

41. Concannon, "Eschatological Implications," 888.

42. Alan Lewis draws attention to this fact: "In the frangibility of bread, so easily disintegrated into crumbs, and in the perilous cup of wine, so readily spilt and lost to human use, we see God's own subjection to the tearing of the flesh, the breaking of bones, the spilling of blood, and the snuffing out of life, which so frequently and tragically" marks our existence today. A. Lewis, *Between Cross and Resurrection*, 396.

43. Lysaught, "Suffering in Communion with Christ," 82.

44. Breckenridge and Vogler, "The Critical Limits of Embodiment."

45. Creamer, *Disability and Christian Theology*, 96.

46. Creamer, *Disability and Christian Theology*, 119.

47. Henson, "Palliative Care's Sacramental and Liturgical Foundations."

48. Lysaught, "Suffering in Communion with Christ," 82n40.

49. The quotation from Saunders is from Clark, *Cicely Saunders*, 122. Quoted in Lysaught, "Suffering in Communion with Christ," 82n40.

50. Henson, "Palliative Care's Sacramental and Liturgical Foundations," 62.

CONCLUSION. Humanity *Sub Specie Mortis*

1. Berry, *Fidelity*. All quotations in this section are from this story unless otherwise noted. Portions of this chapter were originally published in my article, "What's Going on in Canada with Assisted Suicide."
2. Berry, "Health Is Membership," in *Art of the Commonplace*.
3. Berry, "Health Is Membership."
4. Maynard, "My Right to Death with Dignity at 29."
5. See Ziegler, *Wild and Precious Life*. All further quotations in this section regarding Brittany Maynard are from this book.
6. Like Brittany, Kara's story would also have an impact on many people. She was profiled in magazines and news stories, she published two books about her experience, and was featured in a documentary film called *The Long Goodbye*.
7. Tippetts, "Dying with Grace."
8. Email correspondence, November 12, 2013.
9. Email correspondence, November 14, 2013.
10. Murdoch, *Existentialists and Mystics*, 329.
11. For the term "newone," see Mumford, *Ethics at the Beginning of Life*.
12. Interview with Scott and Meg, May 20, 2023.
13. Email correspondence, May 12, 2023.
14. Interview with Scott and Meg, May 20, 2023.
15. Interview with Scott and Meg, May 20, 2023.
16. Journal entry shared with author, March 9, 2014.
17. Journal entry shared with author, March 9, 2014.
18. Interview with Scott and Meg, May 20, 2023.
19. Interview with Scott and Meg, May 20, 2023.
20. Interview with Scott and Meg, May 20, 2023.
21. Interview with Scott and Meg, May 20, 2023.
22. Interview with Scott and Meg, May 20, 2023.

Bibliography

Aquinas, Thomas. *Summa theologiae*. Translated by Michael Rudick. Unpublished text.

———. *Treatise on Law: The Complete Text*. Edited Alfred J. Freddoso. South Bend: St. Augustine's Press, 2009.

Arendt, Hannah. *The Human Condition*. 2nd ed. Chicago: University of Chicago Press, 1998.

Ariès, Philippe. *The Hour of Our Death*. Translated by Helen Weaver. New York: Random House, 1981.

———. *Western Attitudes toward Death: From the Middle Ages to the Present*. London: Marion Boyars, 1976.

Augustine. *Confessions*. Translated by Henry Chadwick. Oxford: Oxford University Press, 2009.

———. *De civitate Dei*. Translated by Marcus Dods. In *Nicene and Post-Nicene Fathers, First Series*. Vol. 2. Edited by Philip Schaff. Buffalo: Christian Literature Publishing, 1887. Revised and edited for New Advent by Kevin Knight.

———. *De vera religione liber unus*. http://www.augustinus.it/latino/vera_religione/.

Banner, Michael. *The Ethics of Everyday Life: Moral Theology, Social Anthropology, and the Imagination of the Human*. Oxford: Oxford University Press, 2014.

———. "Scripts for Modern Dying: The Death before Death We Have Invented, the Death before Death We Fear and Some Take Too Literally, and the Death before Death Christians Believe In." *Studies in Christian Ethics* 29, no. 3 (2016): 249–55.

Barth, Karl. *Christ and Adam: Man and Humanity in Romans 5*. New York: Macmillan, 1968.

———. *Church Dogmatics*. Translated by G. W. Bromiley and T. F. Torrance. Edinburgh: T&T Clark, 1956.

———. *Credo*. New York: Scribner, 1962.

———. *The Epistle to the Romans*. London: Oxford University Press, 1977.

———. *The Humanity of God*. Translated by Thomas Wieser. Atlanta: John Knox Press, 1978.

———. "No!" In *Natural Theology: Comprising "Nature and Grace by Professor Dr. Emil Brunner and the Reply "No!" by Dr. Karl Barth*, translated by Peter Fraenkel, 65–122. London: Centenary Press, 1946.

———. *Wolfgang Amadeus Mozart*. Eugene: Wipf & Stock, 1986.

Battin, Margaret Pabst. *Ending Life: Ethics and the Way We Die*. New York: Oxford University Press, 2005.

Battin, Margaret P., Agnes van der Heide, Linda Ganzini, Gerrit van der Wal, and Bregje D. Onwuteaka-Philipsen. "Legal Physician-Assisted Dying in Oregon and the Netherlands: Evidence concerning the Impact on Patients in 'Vulnerable' Groups." *Journal of Medical Ethics* 33, no. 5 (2007): 591–97.

Bauckham, Richard. *Living with Other Creatures: Green Exegesis and Theology*. Waco: Baylor University Press, 2011.

Bauman, Zygmunt. *Liquid Modernity*. Cambridge: Polity, 2012.

———. *Mortality, Immortality and Other Life Strategies*. Cambridge: Polity, 1992.

———. *Postmodern Ethics*. Oxford: Blackwell, 1993.

Beauchamp, Tom L., and James F. Childress. *Principles of Biomedical Ethics*. 7th ed. New York: Oxford University Press, 2013.

Becker, Ernest. *The Denial of Death*. New York: Free Press, 1973.

———. *The Structure of Evil: An Essay on the Unification of the Science of Man*. New York: George Braziller, 1968.

Bellah, Robert N. *Religion in Human Evolution: From the Paleolithic to the Axial Age*. Cambridge, MA: Harvard University Press, 2011.

Berger, Peter L. *The Sacred Canopy: Elements of a Sociological Theory of Religion*. New York: Anchor Books, 1967.

Berger, Peter L., Brigitte Berger, and Hansfried Kellner. *The Homeless Mind: Modernization and Consciousness*. New York: Random House, 1974.

Berger, Peter L., and Thomas Luckmann. *The Social Construction of Reality: A Treatise in the Sociology of Knowledge*. Garden City, NY: Doubleday, 1966.

Berkouwer, G. C. *The Triumph of Grace in the Theology of Karl Barth*. London: Paternoster Press, 1956.

Berry, Wendell. *The Art of the Commonplace: The Agrarian Essays of Wendell Berry*. Washington, DC: Counterpoint Press, 2002.

———. *Fidelity: Five Stories*. Washington, DC: Counterpoint Press, 2018.

Biggar, Nigel. *The Hastening that Waits: Karl Barth's Ethics*. Oxford: Clarendon, 1993.

Bishop, Jeffrey P. *The Anticipatory Corpse: Medicine, Power, and the Care of the Dying*. Notre Dame: University of Notre Dame Press, 2011.

———. "Finitude." In *Dying in the Twenty-First Century: Toward a New Ethical Framework for the Art of Dying Well*, edited by Lydia Dugdale, 19–32. Cambridge, MA: MIT Press, 2015.

Breckenridge, Carole A., and Candace A. Vogler. "The Critical Limits of Embodiment: Disability's Criticism." *Public Culture* 13, no. 3 (2001): 349–57.

Bregman, Lucy. *Beyond Silence and Denial: Death and Dying Reconsidered*. Louisville: Westminster John Knox, 1994.

Brenan, Megan. "America's Strong Support for Euthanasia Persists." *Gallup News*, May 31, 2018.

Bretzke, James T., S.J. "The Burden of Means: Interpreting Recent Catholic Magisterial Teaching on End-of-Life Issues." *Journal of the Society of Christian Ethics* 26, no. 2 (2006): 183–200.

Brother Lawrence. *The Practice of the Presence of God: Being Conversations and Letters of Nicholas Herman of Lorraine, Brother Lawrence*. Westwood, NJ: Revell, 1958.

Buchbinder, Mara. *Scripting Death: Stories of Assisted Dying in America*. Oakland: University of California Press, 2021.

Burnett, Richard E. *Karl Barth's Theological Exegesis: The Hermeneutical Principles of the* Römerbrief *Period*. Grand Rapids: Eerdmans, 2004.

Burnett, Richard E., ed. *The Westminster Handbook to Karl Barth*. Louisville: Westminster John Knox, 2013.

Burns, John F. "With Help, Conductor and Wife Ended Lives." *New York Times*, July 14, 2009.

Burt, Robert. *Death Is That Man Taking Names: Intersections of American Medicine, Law, and Culture*. Berkeley: University of California Press, 2002.

Busch, Eberhard. *The Great Passion: An Introduction to Karl Barth's Theology*. Translated by Geoffrey Bromiley. Edited by Darrell L. Guder and Judith J. Guder. Grand Rapids: Eerdmans, 2004.

Byock, Ira. *Dying Well: Peace and Possibilities at the End of Life*. New York: Riverhead Books, 1997.

Byock, Ira R., Arthur Caplan, and Lois Snyder. "Beyond Symptom Management: Physician Roles and Responsibility in Palliative Care." In *Physician's Guide to End-of-Life Care*, edited by Lois Snyder and Timothy Quill, 56–71. Philadelphia: American College of Physicians, 2001.

Cahill, Lisa Sowle. "Catholicism, Death, and Modern Medicine." *America*, April 25, 2005, 14–17.

———. "Richard A. McCormick, S.J.,'s 'To Save or Let Die: The Dilemma of Modern Medicine.'" In *The Story of Bioethics: From Seminal Works to Contemporary Explorations*, edited by Jennifer K. Walter and Eran P. Klein, 131–48. Washington, DC: Georgetown University Press, 2003.

Callahan, Daniel. *The Troubled Dream of Life: Living with Mortality.* New York: Simon & Schuster, 1993.

Carter, Stephen L. "Must Liberalism Be Violent? A Reflection on the Work of Stanley Hauerwas." *Law and Contemporary Problems* 75, no. 4 (2012): 201–19.

Cartwright, Michael. "Afterword: Stanley Hauerwas's Essays in Theological Ethics: A Reader's Guide." In *The Hauerwas Reader*, edited by John Berkman and Michael Cartwright, 623–72. Durham, NC: Duke University Press, 2001.

Catechism of the Catholic Church. Vatican City: Libreria Editrice Vaticana, 2003. http://www.vatican.va/archive/ENG0015/_INDEX.HTM.

Cavanaugh, William T. "Killing for the Eucharist or Being Killed by It? Romero's Challenge to First-World Christians." *Theology Today* 58, no. 2 (2001): 177–89.

Childress, James F. "Religious Viewpoints." In *Regulating How We Die: The Ethical, Medical, and Legal Issues Surrounding Physician-Assisted Suicide*, edited by Linda L. Emanuel, 120–50. Cambridge, MA: Harvard University Press, 1998.

Choron, Jacques. *Death and Western Thought.* New York: Collier Books, 1973.

Clark, David. *Cicely Saunders—Founder of the Hospice Movement: Selected Letters, 1959–1999.* New York: Oxford University Press, 2005.

Clough, David. *Ethics in Crisis: Interpreting Barth's Ethics.* Aldershot, UK: Ashgate, 2005.

———. *On Animals: Volume 1 Systematic Theology.* London: T&T Clark, 2012.

Coakley, Sarah. *Powers and Submissions: Spirituality, Philosophy, and Gender.* Oxford: Blackwell, 2002.

———. "Prayer as Crucible: How My Mind Has Changed." *Christian Century*, March 22, 2011, 32–33.

———. "Prayer as Divine Propulsion: An Interview with Sarah Coakley." *The Other Journal* 21 (2012). https://theotherjournal.com/2012/12/prayer-as-divine-propulsion-an-interview-with-sarah-coakley/.

Concannon, Ellen. "The Eschatological Implications of Karl Rahner's Eucharistic Doctrine." *Heythrop Journal* 51 (2010): 881–92.

Congregation for the Doctrine of the Faith. *Declaration on Euthanasia.* Vatican City: Libreria Editrice Vaticana, 2009.

———. "Instruction on Respect for Human Life in Its Origin and on the Dignity of Procreation." February 22, 1987. Vatican City: Libreria Editrice Vaticana, 2009.

Craigo-Snell, Shannon. *Silence, Love, and Death: Saying Yes to God in the Theology of Karl Rahner.* Milwaukee: Marquette University Press, 2008.

Crawford, Matthew B. *Shop Class as Soulcraft: An Inquiry into the Value of Work.* New York: Penguin, 2009.

———. *The World beyond Your Head: On Becoming an Individual in an Age of Distraction.* New York: Farrar, Straus and Giroux, 2015.

Creamer, Deborah Beth. *Disability and Christian Theology: Embodied Limits and Constructive Possibilities.* Oxford: Oxford University Press, 2009.

Dean, Robert J. *For the Life of the World: Jesus Christ and the Church in the Theologies of Dietrich Bonhoeffer and Stanley Hauerwas.* Eugene: Wipf & Stock, 2016.

Deane-Drummond, Celia. *Christ and Evolution: Wonder and Wisdom.* Minneapolis: Fortress Press, 2009.

Deane-Drummond, Celia, and David Clough, eds. *Creaturely Theology: On God, Humans and Other Animals.* London: SCM Press, 2009.

Didion, Joan. *Blue Nights.* New York: Random House, 2011.

———. *The Year of Magical Thinking.* New York: Knopf, 2005.

Dodaro, Robert. *Christ and the Just Society in the Thought of Augustine.* Cambridge: Cambridge University Press, 2004.

Doka, Kenneth J. "The Death Awareness Movement: Description, History, and Analysis." In *Handbook of Death & Dying.* Vol. 1. Edited by Clifton D. Bryant, 50–56. Thousand Oaks: Sage, 2003.

Drought, Theresa, and Barbara Koenig. "'Choice' in End-of-Life Decision Making: Researching Fact or Fiction?" *Gerontologist* 42, no. 3 (2002): 114–28.

Dugdale, Lydia S. *The Lost Art of Dying: Reviving Forgotten Wisdom.* New York: HarperOne, 2020.

Dunlop, Dorothy D., Larry M. Manheim, Jing Song, and Rowland W. Chang. "Gender and Ethnic/Racial Disparities in Health Care Utilization among Older Adults." *Journal of Gerontology: Social Sciences* 57B, no. 3 (2002): S221–33.

Elias, Norbert. *The Loneliness of the Dying.* Oxford: Blackwell, 1985.

Elmhurst, Sophie. "Take Me to the Death Café." *Prospect*, February 2015. https://www.prospectmagazine.co.uk/essays/47104/take-me-to-the-death-cafe.

Emanuel, Ezekiel J. "Four Myths about Doctor-Assisted Suicide." *New York Times*, October 27, 2012.

Feifel, Herman. *The Meaning of Death.* New York: McGraw-Hill, 1965.

———. *New Meanings of Death.* New York: McGraw-Hill, 1977.

Finnis, John. *Moral Absolutes: Tradition, Revision, and Truth.* Washington, DC: Catholic University of America Press, 1991.

Fitts, W.T., Jr., and I. S. Ravdin. "What Philadelphia Physicians Tell Patients with Cancer." *JAMA* 153, no. 10 (1953): 901–4.

Gawande, Atul. *Being Mortal: Medicine and What Matters in the End.* New York: Metropolitan Books, 2014.

———. "Letting Go." *New Yorker*, August 2, 2010.

Gehlen, Arnold. "*Anthropoligische Forschung* (1961)." In *Conservatism: An Anthology of Social and Political Thought from David Hume to the Present*, edited by Jerry Z. Muller, 401–10. Princeton: Princeton University Press, 1997.

Giddens, Anthony. *Modernity and Self-Identity: Self and Society in the Late Modern Age.* Stanford: Stanford University Press, 1991.

Gorer, Geoffrey. "The Pornography of Death." In *Death Grief and Mourning: A Study of Contemporary Society*, 49–52. Garden City, NY: Anchor Books, 1967.

Green, James W. *Beyond the Good Death: The Anthropology of Modern Dying.* Philadelphia: University of Pennsylvania Press, 2008.

Gregory, Brad S. *Salvation at Stake: Christian Martyrdom in Early Modern Europe.* Cambridge, MA: Harvard University Press, 1999.

Grisez, Germaine. *The Way of the Lord Jesus, Volume 1: Christian Moral Principles.* Chicago: Franciscan Herald Press, 1983.

Gustafson, James M. *An Examined Faith: The Grace of Self-Doubt.* Minneapolis: Fortress, 2004.

———. "The Sectarian Temptation: Reflections on Theology, Church and the University." *Proceedings of the Catholic Theological Society* 40 (1985): 83–94.

Guth, Karen. *The Ethics of Tainted Legacies: Human Flourishing after Traumatic Pasts.* Cambridge: Cambridge University Press, 2022.

Haddorff, David W. *Christian Ethics as Witness: Barth's Ethics for a World at Risk.* Eugene: Cascade Books, 2010.

Hafner, Katie. "In Ill Doctor, a Surprise Reflection of Who Picks Assisted Suicide." *New York Times*, August 11, 2012.

Hampson, Daphne. *Theology and Feminism.* Oxford: Blackwell, 1990.

Hanby, Michael. *Augustine and Modernity.* London: Routledge, 2003.

Hancock, Karen, Josephine M. Clayton, Sharon M. Parker, Sharon Walder, Phyllis N. Butow, Sue Carrick, David Currow, Davina Ghersi, Paul Glare, Rebecca Hagerty, and Martin H. N. Tattersall. "Truth-Telling in Discussing Prognosis in Advanced Life-Limiting Illnesses: A Systematic Review." *Palliative Medicine* 21, no. 6 (2007): 507–17.

Hare, John E. *God's Command.* New York: Oxford University Press, 2015.

Harlan, Susan. "My First Name." *South Carolina Review* 49, no. 2 (2017): 101.

Hauerwas, Stanley. *Approaching the End: Eschatological Reflections on Church, Politics, and Life.* Grand Rapids: Eerdmans, 2013.

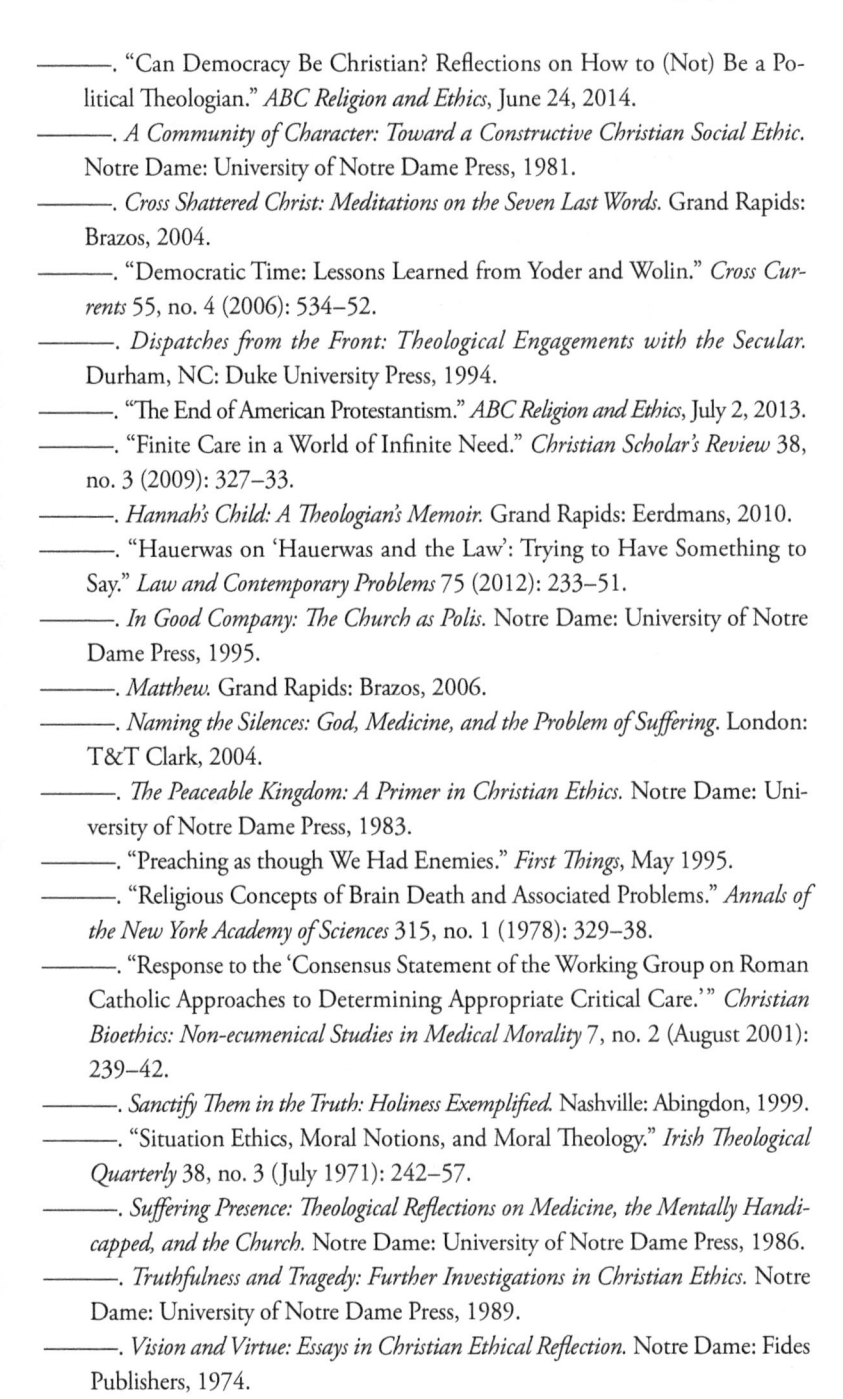

———. "Can Democracy Be Christian? Reflections on How to (Not) Be a Political Theologian." *ABC Religion and Ethics*, June 24, 2014.

———. *A Community of Character: Toward a Constructive Christian Social Ethic*. Notre Dame: University of Notre Dame Press, 1981.

———. *Cross Shattered Christ: Meditations on the Seven Last Words*. Grand Rapids: Brazos, 2004.

———. "Democratic Time: Lessons Learned from Yoder and Wolin." *Cross Currents* 55, no. 4 (2006): 534–52.

———. *Dispatches from the Front: Theological Engagements with the Secular*. Durham, NC: Duke University Press, 1994.

———. "The End of American Protestantism." *ABC Religion and Ethics*, July 2, 2013.

———. "Finite Care in a World of Infinite Need." *Christian Scholar's Review* 38, no. 3 (2009): 327–33.

———. *Hannah's Child: A Theologian's Memoir*. Grand Rapids: Eerdmans, 2010.

———. "Hauerwas on 'Hauerwas and the Law': Trying to Have Something to Say." *Law and Contemporary Problems* 75 (2012): 233–51.

———. *In Good Company: The Church as Polis*. Notre Dame: University of Notre Dame Press, 1995.

———. *Matthew*. Grand Rapids: Brazos, 2006.

———. *Naming the Silences: God, Medicine, and the Problem of Suffering*. London: T&T Clark, 2004.

———. *The Peaceable Kingdom: A Primer in Christian Ethics*. Notre Dame: University of Notre Dame Press, 1983.

———. "Preaching as though We Had Enemies." *First Things*, May 1995.

———. "Religious Concepts of Brain Death and Associated Problems." *Annals of the New York Academy of Sciences* 315, no. 1 (1978): 329–38.

———. "Response to the 'Consensus Statement of the Working Group on Roman Catholic Approaches to Determining Appropriate Critical Care.'" *Christian Bioethics: Non-ecumenical Studies in Medical Morality* 7, no. 2 (August 2001): 239–42.

———. *Sanctify Them in the Truth: Holiness Exemplified*. Nashville: Abingdon, 1999.

———. "Situation Ethics, Moral Notions, and Moral Theology." *Irish Theological Quarterly* 38, no. 3 (July 1971): 242–57.

———. *Suffering Presence: Theological Reflections on Medicine, the Mentally Handicapped, and the Church*. Notre Dame: University of Notre Dame Press, 1986.

———. *Truthfulness and Tragedy: Further Investigations in Christian Ethics*. Notre Dame: University of Notre Dame Press, 1989.

———. *Vision and Virtue: Essays in Christian Ethical Reflection*. Notre Dame: Fides Publishers, 1974.

---. *War and the American Difference: Theological Reflections on Violence and National Identity.* Grand Rapids: Baker Academic, 2011.

---. "What Love Looks Like: Vulnerability, Disability, and the Witness of Jean Vanier." *ABC Religion and Ethics*, March 12, 2015.

---. *Wilderness Wanderings: Probing Twentieth-Century Theology and Philosophy.* London: SCM Press, 2001.

---. *The Work of Theology.* Grand Rapids: Eerdmans, 2015.

---. *Working with Words: On Learning to Speak Christian.* Eugene: Cascade Books, 2011.

Hauerwas, Stanley, and Richard Bondi. "Memory, Community, and the Reasons for Living: Reflections on Suicide and Euthanasia (1976)." In *The Hauerwas Reader*, edited by John Berkman and Michael Cartwright, 577–95. Durham, NC: Duke University Press, 2001.

Hauerwas, Stanley, and David Burrell. "From System to Story: An Alternative Pattern for Rationality in Ethics." In *Truthfulness and Tragedy: Further Investigations in Christian Ethics*, 15–39. South Bend: University of Notre Dame Press, 1977.

Hauerwas, Stanley, and Gerry McKenney. "Doing Nothing Gallantly." In *Approaching the End: Eschatological Reflections on Church, Politics, and Life*, 200–221. Grand Rapids: Eerdmans, 2013.

Hauerwas, Stanley, and Charles Pinches. "Practicing Patience: How Christians Should Be Sick (1997)." In *The Hauerwas Reader*, edited by John Berkman and Michael Cartwright, 348–70. Durham, NC: Duke University Press, 2001.

---. "Witness." In *Approaching the End: Eschatological Reflections on Church, Politics, and Life*, 37–63. Grand Rapids: Eerdmans, 2013.

Hauerwas, Stanley, and Jean Vanier. *Living Gently in a Violent World: The Prophetic Witness of Weakness.* Downers Grove, IL: IVP Books, 2008.

Hawkins, Jennifer S., and Ezekiel Emanuel. "Clarifying Confusions about Coercion." *Hastings Center Report* 35, no. 5 (2005): 16–19.

Hays, Richard B. Foreword to *The Difference Christ Makes: Celebrating the Life, Work, and Friendship of Stanley Hauerwas*, ix–x. Edited by Charles Collier. Eugene: Wipf & Stock, 2015.

Heidegger, Martin. *Being and Time: A Translation of Sein und Zeit.* Translated by Joan Stambaugh. Albany: State University of New York Press, 1996.

---. *The Fundamental Concepts of Metaphysics: World, Finitude, Solitude.* Bloomington: Indiana University Press, 1995.

Henson, Darren M. "Palliative Care's Sacramental and Liturgical Foundations: Healthcare Formed by Faith, Hope, and Love." PhD diss., Marquette University, 2014.

Hitchens, Christopher. *Mortality.* New York: Twelve, 2012.
Hockey, Jennifer. *Experiences of Death: An Anthropological Account.* Edinburgh: Edinburgh University Press, 1990.
Holton, Richard. "Memory, Persons, Dementia." *Studies in Christian Ethics* 29, no. 3 (2016): 256–60.
Hovey, Craig. *To Share in the Body: A Theology of Martyrdom for Today's Church.* Grand Rapids: Brazos, 2008.
Huebner, Chris K. *A Precarious Peace: Yoderian Exploration on Theology, Knowledge and Identity.* Scottsdale: Herald Press, 2006.
Humphry, Derek. *Final Exit: The Practicalities of Self-Deliverance and Assisted Suicide for the Dying.* 3rd ed. New York: Delta, 2002.
Hunsinger, George. *How to Read Karl Barth: The Shape of His Theology.* New York: Oxford University Press, 1991.
———. *Reading Barth with Charity: A Hermeneutical Proposal.* Grand Rapids: Baker Academic, 2015.
———. "The Yes Hidden in Barth's No to Brunner: The First Commandment as a Theological Axiom." In *Evangelical, Catholic, and Reformed: Doctrinal Essays on Barth and Related Themes*, 85–105. Grand Rapids: Eerdmans, 2015.
Illich, Ivan. *Medical Nemesis: The Expropriation of Health.* New York: Pantheon, 1976.
Irenaeus. *Against Heresies.* Translated by Alexander Roberts and William Rambaut. In *Ante-Nicene Fathers.* Vol. 1. Edited by Alexander Roberts, James Donaldson, and A. Cleveland Coxe, 309–567. Buffalo: Christian Literature Publishing, 1885. Revised and edited for New Advent by Kevin Knight.
John Paul II. *Address to the Participants in the International Congress on "Life-Sustaining Treatments and Vegetative State: Scientific Advances and Ethical Dilemmas."* March 2004. Vatican City: Libreria Editrice Vaticana, 2009.
———. *Evangelium Vitae, Encyclical Letter.* Vatican City: Libreria Editrice Vaticana, 2009.
———. *Love and Responsibility.* Rev. ed. New York: Farrar, Straus and Giroux, 1981.
———. *Reconciliatio et Paenitentia: Apostolic Exhortation.* Vatican City: Libreria Editrice Vaticana, 2009.
———. *Veritatis Splendor, Encyclical Letter.* Vatican City: Libreria Editrice Vaticana, 2009.
Jones, David Albert. *Approaching the End: A Theological Exploration of Death and Dying.* Oxford: Oxford University Press, 2007.
Jotkowitz A. B., and S. Glick. "The Groningen Protocol: Another Perspective." *Journal of Medical Ethics* 32, no. 3 (2006): 157–58.
Joyce, Adam. "You Always Begin an Essay (or a Theology) in the Middle: A Review of Stanley Hauerwas's *The Work of Theology*." *The Other Journal*, April 13, 2016.

https://theotherjournal.com/2016/04/always-begin-essay-theology-middle-review-stanley-hauerwass-work-theology/.

Kalanithi, Paul. *When Breath Becomes Air.* New York: Random House, 2016.

Kallenberg, Brad. *Ethics as Grammar: Changing the Postmodern Subject.* Notre Dame: University of Notre Dame Press, 2001.

Kaltwasser, Cambria. "The Measure of Our Days: Assessing the Aims of Radical Life Extension in Conversation with Karl Barth's Theology of Human Temporality." Paper presented at the Annual Meeting of the American Academy of Religion, November 22, 2014.

Kapic, Kelly M., and Bruce L. McCormack, eds. *Mapping Modern Theology: A Thematic and Historical Introduction.* Grand Rapids: Baker Academic, 2012.

Kaufman, Sharon R. *And a Time to Die: How American Hospitals Shape the End of Life.* New York: Scribner, 2005.

———. *Ordinary Medicine: Extraordinary Treatments, Longer Lives, and Where to Draw the Line.* Durham, NC: Duke University Press, 2015.

Kelsey, David H. *Eccentric Existence: A Theological Anthropology.* Louisville: Westminster John Knox, 2009.

———. "Two Theologies of Death: Anthropological Gleanings." *Modern Theology* 13, no. 3 (July 1997): 347–70.

Kerr, Fergus. *Immortal Longings: Versions of Transcending Humanity.* Notre Dame: University of Notre Dame Press, 1997.

Kerr, Nathan R. *Christ, History and Apocalyptic: The Politics of Christian Mission.* Eugene: Cascade Books, 2008.

Kierkegaard, Søren. "At a Graveside." In *Three Discourses on Imagined Occasions*, translated by Howard and Edna Hong, 69–102. Princeton: Princeton University Press, 1993.

———. *The Concept of Anxiety: A Simple Psychologically Orienting Deliberation on the Dogmatic Issue of Hereditary Sin.* Princeton: Princeton University Press, 1980.

———. *The Sickness unto Death: A Christian Psychological Exposition for Edification and Awakening by Anti-climacus.* London: Penguin, 1989.

———. *Works of Love: Some Christian Reflections in the Form of Discourses.* London: Collins, 1962.

Kübler-Ross, Elisabeth. *On Death and Dying.* New York: Macmillan, 1969.

Latkovic, Mark. "Moral Theology: A Survey." In *Encyclopedia of Catholic Social Thought, Social Science, and Social Policy.* Vol. 2. Edited by Michael L Coulter, 716–20. Lanham: Scarecrow, 2007.

Le Pichon, Xavier. "The Sign of Contradiction." In *The Paradox of Disability: Responses to Jean Vanier and L'Arche Communities from Theology and the Sciences*, edited by Hans Reinders, 94–100. Grand Rapids: Eerdmans, 2010.

Lewis, Alan E. *Between Cross and Resurrection: A Theology of Holy Saturday.* Grand Rapids: Eerdmans, 2001.
Lewis, C. S. "Membership." In *The Weight of Glory: And Other Addresses*, 158–76. New York: HarperCollins, 2000.
———. *Mere Christianity.* San Francisco: Harper, 2001.
Lindemann, Hilde. *Holding and Letting Go: The Social Practice of Personal Identities.* Oxford: Oxford University Press, 2014.
Lindemann, Hilde, and Marian Verkerk. "Ending the Life of a Newborn: The Groningen Protocol." *Hastings Center Report* 38, no. 1 (2008): 42–51.
Lustig, Andrew. "Prescribing Prayer?" *Commonweal Magazine*, May 12, 2004.
Lysaught, M. Therese. "Suffering in Communion with Christ: Sacraments, Dying Faithfully, and End-of-Life Care." In *Living Well and Dying Faithfully: Christian Practices for End-of-Life Care*, edited by John Swinton and Richard Payne, 59–85. Grand Rapids: Eerdmans, 2009.
———. "Witnessing Christ in Their Bodies: Martyrs and Ascetics as Doxological Disciples." *Annual of the Society of Christian Ethics* 20 (2000): 239–62.
MacKendrick, Kenneth G. "Intersubjectivity and the Revival of Death: Toward a Critique of Sovereign Individualism." *Critical Sociology* 31, no. 1–2 (2005): 169–83.
Mangina, Joseph. *Karl Barth: Theologian of Christian Witness.* Louisville: Westminster John Knox, 2004.
Mantwill, S., S. Monestel-Umaña, and P. J. Schulz. "The Relationship between Health Literacy and Health Disparities: A Systematic Review." *PLoS ONE* 10, no. 12 (2015): e0145455.
Mathewes, Charles T. "Augustinian Anthropology: Interior *Intimo Meo.*" *Journal of Religious Ethics* 27, no. 2 (1999): 195–221.
Mauceri, Joseph M. "Euthanasia." In *Encyclopedia of Catholic Social Thought, Social Science, and Social Policy.* Vol. 1. Edited by Michael L. Coulter, 377–78. Lanham: Scarecrow, 2007.
May, William E. *An Introduction to Moral Theology.* 2nd ed. Huntington, IN: Our Sunday Visitor, 2003.
Maynard, Brittany. "My Right to Death with Dignity at 29." *CNN*, October 7, 2014. https://www.cnn.com/2014/10/07/opinion/maynard-assisted-suicide-cancer-dignity/index.html.
McCarty, Brett. "Diagnosis and Therapy in *The Anticipatory Corpse*: A Second Opinion." *Journal of Medicine and Philosophy* 41 (2016): 621–41.
McCormack, Bruce L. *Karl Barth's Critically Realistic Dialectical Theology: Its Genesis and Development, 1909–1936.* Oxford: Oxford University Press, 1997.
———. *Orthodox and Modern: Studies in the Theology of Karl Barth.* Grand Rapids: Baker Academic, 2008.

McCormick, Richard A., S.J. "The Consistent Ethic of Life: Is There a Historical Soft Underbelly?" In *The Critical Calling: Reflections on Moral Dilemmas since Vatican II*, 211–32. Washington, DC: Georgetown University Press, 1989.

———. *Health and Medicine in the Catholic Tradition: Tradition in Transition*. New York: Crossroad Publishing, 1984.

———. *How Brave a New World? Dilemmas in Bioethics*. Garden City, NY: Doubleday, 1981.

———. "Killing the Patient." In *Considering Veritatis Splendor*, edited by John Wilkins, 14–20. Cleveland: Pilgrim Press, 1994.

———. "Letter to the Editor." *Hastings Center Report* 5, no. 2 (1975): 4.

———. "Notes on Moral Theology: April–September 1972: Of Death and Dying." *Theological Studies* 34, no. 1 (1973): 65–77.

———. "Physician-Assisted Suicide: Flight from Compassion." *Christian Century*, December 4, 1991, 1132–34.

———. "The Consistent Ethic of Life: Is There a Historical Soft Underbelly?" In *The Critical Calling: Reflections on Moral Dilemmas since Vatican II*, 211–32. Washington, DC: Georgetown University Press, 1989.

———. "The Quality of Life, the Sanctity of Life." *Hastings Center Report* 8, no. 1 (1978): 30–36.

———. "Theology and Bioethics." *Hastings Center Report* 19, no. 2 (1989): 5–10.

———. "To Save or Let Die: The Dilemma of Modern Medicine." *Journal of the American Medical Association* 229, no. 2 (1974): 172–76.

McDowell, John C. "Much Ado about Nothing: Karl Barth's Being Unable to Do Nothing about Nothingness." *International Journal of Systematic Theology* 4, no. 3 (2002): 319–35.

McGill, Arthur C. *Death and Life: An American Theology*. Eugene: Wipf & Stock, 2003.

McKenny, Gerald P. *The Analogy of Grace: Karl Barth's Moral Theology*. Oxford: Oxford University Press, 2010.

Medley, Mark S. "'Always Carrying in the Body the Death of Jesus': Baptism, Martyrdom, and Quotidian Existence in Rowan Williams' Theology." *Anglican Theological Review* 94, no. 3 (2012): 475–93.

Meilaender, Gilbert. "Euthanasia & Christian Vision." *Thought* 57 (1982): 465–75.

———. "I Want to Burden My Loved Ones." *First Things* 16 (October 1991): 12–16.

———. *Should We Live Forever? The Ethical Ambiguities of Aging*. Grand Rapids: Eerdmans, 2013.

Merkle, Judith A. "Personalism." In *The New Dictionary of Catholic Social Thought*, edited by Judith A. Dwyer, 737–38. Collegeville, MN: Liturgical Press, 1994.

Migliore, Daniel L. *Commanding Grace: Studies in Karl Barth's Ethics*. Grand Rapids: Eerdmans, 2010.

Milbank, John. "Sacred Triads: Augustine and the Indo-European Soul." In *Augustine and His Critics: Essays in Honor of Gerald Bonner*, edited by Robert Dodaro and George Lawless, 77–102. London: Routledge, 2000.

Mitford, Jessica. *The American Way of Death*. New York: Simon & Schuster, 1963.

———. *The American Way of Death Revisited*. New York: Knopf, 1998.

Modras, Ronald. "The Thomistic Personalism of Pope John Paul II." *Modern Schoolman* 59 (1982): 117–27.

Moltmann, Jürgen. *God in Creation: An Ecological Doctrine of Creation: The Gifford Lectures 1984–1985*. London: SCM Press, 1985.

Moore, Stephen, ed. *Divinanimality: Animal Theory, Creaturely Theology*. New York: Fordham University Press, 2014.

Moyse, Ashley. *Resourcing Hope for Ageing and Dying in a Broken World: Wayfaring through Despair*. New York: Anthem, 2022.

Mulhall, Stephen. *Philosophical Myths of the Fall*. Princeton: Princeton University Press, 2005.

Mumford, James. *Ethics at the Beginning of Life: A Phenomenological Critique*. Oxford: Oxford University Press, 2013.

———. *Vexed: Ethics beyond Political Tribes*. London: Bloomsbury, 2020.

Murdoch, Iris. *Existentialists and Mystics*. Harmondsworth, UK: Penguin, 1997.

———. *The Sovereignty of Good*. London: Routledge, 2001.

Nakashima, George. *The Soul of a Tree: A Woodworker's Reflections*. Tokyo: Kodansha, 1988.

Niebuhr, H. Richard. "The Grace of Doing Nothing." *Christian Century* 49 (March 23, 1932): 378–80.

Niebuhr, Reinhold. "Must We Do Nothing?" *Christian Century* 49 (March 30, 1932): 415–17.

———. *The Nature and Destiny of Man: A Christian Interpretation*. New York: Scribner, 1964.

Nimmo, Paul T. *Being in Action: The Theological Shape of Barth's Ethical Vision*. London: T&T Clark, 2007.

Norwood, Frances, Gerrit Kimsma, and Margaret P. Battin. "Vulnerability and the 'Slippery Slope' at the End-of-Life: A Qualitative Study of Euthanasia, General Practice and Home Death in the Netherlands." *Family Practice* 26, no. 6 (2009): 472–80.

Nuland, Sherwin. *How We Die: Reflections On Life's Final Chapter.* New York: Knopf, 1993.

Nussbaum, Abraham M. *The Finest Traditions of My Calling: One Physician's Search for the Renewal of Medicine.* New Haven: Yale University Press, 2016.

Ochs, Robert. "Death as Act: An Interpretation of Karl Rahner." In *The Mystery of Suffering and Death,* edited by Michael J. Taylor, 119–38. New York: Alba House, 1973.

Osborn, Ronald E. *Death before the Fall: Biblical Literalism and the Problem of Animal Suffering.* Downers Grove, IL: IVP Academic, 2014.

Pelikan, Jaroslav. *The Shape of Death: Life, Death, and Immortality in the Early Fathers.* Westport, CT: Greenwood, 1978.

Pendergast, T. J., and J. M. Luce. "Increasing Incidence of Withholding and Withdrawal of Life Support from the Critically Ill." *American Journal of Respiratory Critical Care Medicine* 155, no. 1 (1997): 15–20.

Pereira, J. "Legalizing Euthanasia or Assisted Suicide: The Illusion of Safeguards and Controls." *Current Oncology* 18, no. 2 (2011): 38–45.

Phan, Peter C. "Eschatology." In *The Cambridge Companion to Karl Rahner,* edited by Declan Marmion and Mary E. Hines, 174–92. New York: Cambridge University Press, 2005.

Pickell, Travis. "Gentle Space-Making: Christian Silent Prayer, Mindfulness, and Kenotic Identity Formation." *Studies in Christian Ethics* 32, no. 1 (2019): 66–77.

———. "The Phenomenon of Burdened Agency." *Journal of the Society of Christian Ethics* 44, no. 1 (2024).

———. "What's Going on in Canada with Assisted Suicide? MAID, Moral Imagination, and the Challenge of a Common Good Bioethics." *Church Life Journal.* January 12, 2024. https://churchlifejournal.nd.edu/articles/whats-going-on-in-canada-with-assisted-suicide/

Pinckaers, Servais. *The Spirituality of Martyrdom . . . To the Limits of Love.* Washington, DC: Catholic University of America Press, 2016.

Pius XII. *Acta Apostalicae Sedis* 49 (1957). Vatican City: Libreria Editrice Vaticana, 2009.

Puffer, Matthew. "Taking Exception to the *Grenzfall*'s Reception: Revisiting Karl Barth's Ethics of War." *Modern Theology* 28, no. 3 (July 2012): 478–502.

Putnam, Constance E. *Hospice or Hemlock? Searching for Heroic Compassion.* Westport, CT: Praeger, 2002.

Quill, Timothy. "Death and Dignity—a Case of Individualized Decision Making." *New England Journal of Medicine* 324 (1991): 691–94.

———. *A Midwife through the Dying Process: Stories of Healing and Hard Choices at the End of Life.* Baltimore: Johns Hopkins University Press, 1996.

Rahner, Karl, S.J. "The Eucharist and Our Daily Lives." *Theological Investigations* 7 (1962): 211–26.

———. "On Christian Dying." In *Theological Investigations*. Vol. 7. Translated by David Bourke, 285–93. New York: Seabury, 1971.

———. *On the Theology of Death*. 2nd ed. Freiburg: Herder and Herder, 1965.

Raikin, Alexander. "No Other Options." *New Atlantis* (Winter 2023). https://www.thenewatlantis.com/publications/no-other-options.

Ramsey, Paul. *Ethics at the Edges of Life: Medical and Legal Intersections*. New Haven: Yale University Press, 1978.

———. "Liturgy and Ethics." *Journal of Religious Ethics* 7, no. 2 (1979): 139–71.

———. *The Patient as Person: Explorations in Medical Ethics*. 2nd ed. New Haven: Yale University Press, 2002.

Rawls, John. *A Theory of Justice*. Rev. ed. Cambridge, MA: Belknap, 1999.

Reiser, Stanley Joel. *Medicine and the Reign of Technology*. New York: Cambridge University Press, 1978.

Remenyi, Matthias. "Death as the Limit to Life and Thought: A Thanatological Outline." Translated by Alex Holznienkemper. *Heythrop Journal* 55 (2014): 94–109.

Reuther, Rosemary Radford. "The Left Hand of God in the Theology of Karl Barth: Karl Barth as a Mythopoetic Theologian." *Journal of Religious Thought* 25 (1968–69): 3–26.

———. *Sexism and God-Talk*. London: SCM Press, 1983.

Ridenour, Autumn Alcott. "The Coming of Age: Curse or Calling? Toward a Christological Interpretation of Aging as Call in the Theology of Karl Barth and W. H. Vanstone." *Journal of the Society of Christian Ethics* 33, no. 2 (Fall/Winter 2013): 151–67.

Risse, Guenter B. *Mending Bodies, Saving Souls: A History of Hospitals*. Oxford: Oxford University Press, 1999.

Rogers, Eugene F., Jr. "Theology in the Curriculum of a Secular Religious Studies Department." *Cross Currents* 56, no. 2 (2006): 169–79.

Rose, Matthew. *Ethics with Barth: God, Metaphysics, and Morals*. Farnham, UK: Ashgate, 2010.

Rourke, Thomas. "Personalism." In *Encyclopedia of Catholic Social Thought, Social Science, and Social Policy*. Vol. 2. Edited by Michael L. Coulter, 801–3. Lanham: Scarecrow, 2007.

Ryan, Maura A. *Ethics and Economics of Assisted Reproduction: The Cost of Longing*. Washington, DC: Georgetown University Press, 2001.

Sandel, Michael J. "The Procedural Republic and the Unencumbered Self." *Political Theory* 12, no. 1 (1984): 81–96.

———. *What Money Can't Buy: The Moral Limits of Markets*. New York: Farrar, Straus and Giroux, 2012.

Schleiermacher, Friedrich. *The Christian Faith*. Philadelphia: Fortress, 1976.

———. *On the* Glaubenslehre*: Two Letters to Dr. Lücke*. Translated by James Duke and Francis Fiorenza. American Academy of Religion Texts and Translation Series 3. Chico: Scholars Press, 1981.

Schwartz, Barry. *The Paradox of Choice: Why More Is Less*. New York: ECCO, 2004.

Shavelson, Lonny. *A Chosen Death: The Dying Confront Assisted Suicide*. New York: Simon & Schuster, 1995.

Sherman, Robert. *The Shift to Modernity: Christ and the Doctrine of Creation in the Theologies of Schleiermacher and Barth*. New York: T&T Clark, 2005.

Singer, Peter. *Practical Ethics*. 2nd ed. New York: Cambridge University Press, 1993.

Sonderegger, Katherine. "Creation." In *Mapping Modern Theology: A Thematic and Historical Introduction*, edited by Kelly M. Kapic and Bruce L. McCormack, 97–120. Grand Rapids: Baker Academic, 2012.

Soto, Graciela J., Greg S. Martin, and Michelle Ng Gong. "Healthcare Disparities in Critical Illness." *Critical Care Medicine* 41, no. 12 (2013): 2784–93.

Stout, Jeffrey. *Democracy and Tradition*. Princeton: Princeton University Press, 2004.

———. *Ethics after Babel: The Languages of Morals and Their Discontents*. Boston: Beacon, 1988.

Sulmasy, Daniel. "Transcript of IQ2 Debate: Legalize Assisted Suicide?" (2014). https://opentodebate.org/debate/legalize-assisted-suicide/.

Swinton, John. *Dementia: Living in the Memories of God*. Grand Rapids: Eerdmans, 2012.

Tanner, Kathryn. "Creation and Providence." In *The Cambridge Companion to Karl Barth*, edited by John B. Webster, 111–26. Cambridge: Cambridge University Press, 2000.

Taylor, Charles. *The Ethics of Authenticity*. Cambridge, MA: Harvard University Press, 1991.

———. *Modern Social Imaginaries*. Durham, NC: Duke University Press, 2004.

———. *A Secular Age*. Cambridge, MA: Belknap, 2007.

———. *Sources of the Self: The Making of the Modern Identity*. Cambridge, MA: Harvard University Press, 1989.

Taylor, J. S. "On Recognition, Caring and Dementia." *Medical Anthropology Quarterly* 22, no. 4 (2008): 313–35.

Tessman, Lisa. *Burdened Virtues: Virtue Ethics for Liberatory Struggles*. New York: Oxford University Press, 2005.

The, A.-M., T. Hak, G. Koeter, and G. van der Wal. "Collusion in Doctor-Patient Communication about Imminent Death: An Ethnographic Study." *BMJ* 321 (2000): 1376–81.

Tillich, Paul. *Systematic Theology, Volume 2: Existence and the Christ*. Chicago: University of Chicago Press, 1957.

Tippetts, Kara. "Dying with Grace: An Interview with Kara Tippetts." *byFaith*, March 23, 2015. https://byfaithonline.com/dying-with-grace/.

Tollefson, Christopher. "Does God Intend Death?" *Diametros* 38 (2013): 191–200.

———. "The New Natural Law Theory." *Lyceum* 10, no. 1 (2008): 1–17.

Tolstoy, Leo. *The Death of Ivan Ilyich*. Translated by Lynn Solotaroff. New York: Bantam Dell, 2004.

Toole, David. *Waiting for Godot in Sarajevo: Theological Reflections on Nihilism, Tragedy, and Apocalypse*. Boulder: Westview, 1998.

Townes, Emilie Maureen. *Breaking the Fine Rain of Death: African American Health Issues and a Womanist Ethic of Care*. New York: Continuum, 1998.

Tully, Patrick Andrew. *Refined Consequentialism: The Moral Theory of Richard A. McCormick*. New York: Peter Lang, 2006.

United States Conference of Catholic Bishops. *Ethical and Religious Directives for Catholic Health Care Services*, 5th ed. Washington, DC: United States Conference of Bishops, 2009. http://www.usccb.org/issues-and-action/human-life-and-dignity/health-care/upload/Ethical-Religious-Directives-Catholic-Health-Care-Services-fifth-edition-2009.pdf.

Van Driel, Edwin Christian. *Incarnation Anyway: Arguments for Supralapsarian Christology*. Oxford: Oxford University Press, 2008.

Vanstone, W. H. *The Stature of Waiting*. London: Darton, Longman and Todd, 2004.

Velleman, J. David. "Against the Right to Die." *Journal of Medicine and Philosophy* 17, no. 6 (1992): 665–81.

Verhey, Allen. *The Christian Art of Dying: Learning from Jesus*. Grand Rapids: Eerdmans, 2011.

Verhey, Allen, and Brett McCarty. "The Virtues of Dying Well." *Christian Reflection* (2013): 26–33.

Wailoo, Keith. *Drawing Blood: Technology and Disease Identity in Twentieth-Century America*. Baltimore: Johns Hopkins University Press, 1999.

———. *Dying in the City of the Blues: Sickle Cell Anemia and the Politics of Race and Health*. Chapel Hill: University of North Carolina Press, 2001.

———. *How Cancer Crossed the Color Line*. Oxford: Oxford University Press, 2011.

Wailoo, Keith, and Stephen Gregory Pemberton. *The Troubled Dream of Genetic Medicine: Ethnicity and Innovation in Tay-Sachs, Cystic Fibrosis, and Sickle Cell Disease*. Baltimore: Johns Hopkins University Press, 2006.

Walter, Tony. "Facing Death without Tradition." In *Contemporary Issues in the Sociology of Death, Dying and Disposal*, edited by Glennys Howarth and Peter Jupp, 193–204. London: Macmillan, 1996.

Wannenwetsch, Berndt. "Loving the Limit: Dietrich Bonhoeffer's Hermeneutic of Human Creatureliness and Its Challenge for an Ethics of Medical Care." In *Bonhoeffer and the Biosciences: An Initial Exploration*, edited by R. Wüstenberg, Stefan Heuser, and Esther Hornung, 89–108. New York: Peter Lang, 2009.

Ward, Graham. "Suffering and Incarnation." In *Suffering Religion*, edited by Robert Gibbs and Elliot R. Wolfson, 163–80. London: Routledge, 2002.

Wasson, Katherine, Eva Bading, John Hardt, Lena Hatchett, Mark G. Kuczewski, Michael McCarthy, Aaron Michelfelder, and Kayhan Parsi. "Physician, Know Thyself: The Role of Reflection in Bioethics and Professionalism Education." *Narrative Inquiry in Bioethics* 5, no. 1 (2015): 77–86.

Weber, Max. *From Max Weber: Essays in Sociology*. London: Routledge, 2001.

———. *The Protestant Ethic and the Spirit of Capitalism*. 3rd ed. Los Angeles: Roxbury, 2002.

Webster, John B. *Barth's Moral Theology: Human Action in Barth's Thought*. Edinburgh: T&T Clark, 1998.

Werpehowski, William. *Karl Barth and Christian Ethics: Living in Truth*. Aldershot, UK: Ashgate, 2014.

Westphal, Merold. "Prayer as the Posture of the Decentered Self." In *The Phenomenology of Prayer*, edited by Bruce Ellis Benson and Norman Wirzba, 13–31. New York: Fordham University Press, 2005.

Wicker, Brian. "Conflict and Martyrdom after 11 September 2001." *Theology* 106 (2003): 159–67.

———. "The Drama of Martyrdom: Christian and Muslim Approaches." In *Witnesses to Faith? Martyrdom in Christianity and Islam*, edited by Brian Wicker, 105–16. Burlington, VT: Ashgate, 2006.

Williams, David R., and Pamela Braboy Jackson. "Social Sources of Racial Disparities in Health." *Health Affairs* 24, no. 2 (2005): 325–34.

Williams, Rowan. *On Christian Theology*. Oxford: Blackwell, 1999.

———. *Resurrection: Interpreting the Easter Gospel*. Harrisburg, PA: Morehouse, 1994.

———. *Tokens of Trust: An Introduction to Christian Belief*. London: Canterbury Press Norwich, 2007.

Wojtyła, Karol. *The Acting Person*. Translated by Andrzej Potocki. Edited by Anna-Teresa Tymieniecka. Dordrecht: Reidel, 1979.

Wolterstorff, Nicholas. "Barth on Evil." *Faith and Philosophy* 13 (1996): 584–608.

Wordsworth, William. *The Prelude: Or Growth of a Poet's Mind*. Edited by Ernest De Selincourt. Cambridge: Chadwyck-Healey, 1994.

Yoder, John Howard. *The Politics of Jesus: Vicit Agnus Noster*. Grand Rapids: Eerdmans, 1972.

Ziegler, Deborah. *Wild and Precious Life*. New York: Emily Bestler Books, 2016.

Index

A
Arendt, Hannah, 155n.58
Aries, Philippe, 7–8
ars moriendi, 7
apocalyptic. *See* eschatology
Aquinas, Thomas
   on mortality, 41
   souls and bodies in heaven, 159n.4
Augustine of Hippo
   on Eucharist, 125
   — and reverse metabolism, 178n.39
   on interiority, 30, 158n.38
   on martyrdom, 59
   timor mortis, 155n.58

B
Bacon, Francis
   Baconian project, 63
   science as control of nature, 34
Banner, Michael
   on "death before death," 122–23
   on scripts for dying, 22, 27
   — commonalities between, 37
   — as lived out, 142
baptism
   connected to martyrdom, 121
   dying and rising with Christ, 120
   and eccentric identity, 122
   remembrance of, 123–24
   and surrender, 123
   symbolism of, 119–20
Barth, Karl, xviii
   actualistic ontology, 67, 167n.13
   on Adam, 74–75, 78–79
   Christocentrism, 66
   creaturely finitude, 63, 77–80, 86
   death as sign of judgment, 69–70
   divine command ethic, 81
   doctrine of creation, 61–62
   — and chaos, 167n.12
   embracing finitude, 81–84
   empirical death, 64–66
   ethics as correspondence, 81
   evil (*das Nichtige*), 66–69
   Grenzfall (boundary case), 169n.32
   infinite qualitative distinction, 71, 73
   on Jesus's death, 73, 76–77
   Kant's influence on, 168n.27
   line of death (*Todeslinie*), 71–74
   Mozart, 68, 168n.15
   natural death, 63–64, 75–77
   receptive agency, 84–86
   respect for life, 83–84

Barth, Karl (*cont.*)
  Romans commentary, 70–74
  supralapsarianism, 67, 77
Battin, Margaret, on Stoic (active) vs. Christian (passive) dying, 39, 58
Bauman, Zigmunt, 18, 112, 155n.62
Becker, Ernest, 16–17
Bellah, Robert, 154n.50
Berger, Peter, 15–16
Berry, Wendell
  "Fidelity," 132–37
biblical references
  Genesis 1:24–31, 78
  Genesis 3:19, 79
  Genesis 3:22, 74–75
  Numbers 23:10, 76
  Deuteronomy 31:8, 145
  2 Samuel 14:14, 64
  1 Kings 2:3, 76
  Job 2:9, 144
  Job 2:11–13, 144
  Job 7:9, 64
  Job 16:22, 64
  Psalm 6:3, 65
  Psalm 22:29, 79
  Psalm 30:9, 63, 79
  Psalm 88:11–12, 63
  Psalm 115:17, 63
  Isaiah 38:18–19, 63
  Matthew 16:25, 63
  Matthew 20:22–23, 120
  Matthew 26:26–28, 124
  Matthew 27:46, 70
  Mark 10:38–39, 120
  Mark 12:28–31, 49
  Luke 12:50, 120
  Luke 22:19–20, 124
  Luke 22:42, 126
  John 6:33, 125
  John 6:53–58, 125
  John 12:24, 63
  John 13:34, 49
  John 20:24–28, 114
  John 20:27, 128
  Acts 22:16, 120
  Romans 3:8, 44
  Romans 5:8, 113
  Romans 6:3–5, 120
  Romans 6:6–14, 57
  Romans 6:8, 57
  Romans 7:4–6, 57
  Romans 8:2, 57
  Romans 8:6–12, 57
  Romans 8:17, 126
  Romans 8:29, 128
  Romans 8:34, 113
  Romans 12:5, 127
  Galatians 2:19, 127
  Galatians 3:13, 113
  Galatians 6:2, 145
  Galatians 6:17, 126
  Ephesians 3:6, 127
  Ephesians 4:5, 120
  Ephesians 4:15, 128
  Ephesians 5:2, 113
  Ephesians 5:23, 127
  Philippians 3:10, 127
  Colossians 1:18–24, 127
  Colossians 2:11–12, 120
  1 Corinthians 11:28, 124
  1 Corinthians 12:13, 120
  1 Corinthians 12:27, 127
  1 Corinthians 15:17–19, 114
  1 Corinthians 15:18, 57
  1 Corinthians 15:31, 126

1 Corinthians 15:45, 63
2 Corinthians 1:5–11, 126
2 Corinthians 3:18, 128
2 Corinthians, 4:8–11, 127
2 Corinthians 5:17, 120
2 Corinthians 13:4, 127
1 Thessalonians 4:13–18, 57
1 Thessalonians 5:10, 113
2 Timothy 2:11, 57
Titus 2:14, 113
Hebrews 9:27, 42
Hebrews 10:31, 69
1 John 3:16, 113
Revelation 7:17, 126
Revelation 13:8, 126
Bishop, Jeffrey, on medicine's epistemology, 9–10
Book of Common Prayer, 111
burdened agency
  in Berry's "Fidelity," 132–37
  burden *of* agency, 10–12
  and creaturely finitude, 86
  defined, xiii–xiv, 3–5, 19
  and modern identity, 35–38
  product of expectations, 99

C

Cahill, Lisa, 50
Callahan, Daniel, 27
  on technological brinkmanship, 11
Catechism of the Catholic Church
  on death and dying, 40–44
  on moral objects, 49
  on suicide, 43–44
  on withdrawal of treatment, 43
Cavanaugh, William, 125
Cavell, Stanley, 62
Cloud of Unknowing, 115–17

Coakley, Sarah
  on Lord's prayer, 148–49
  response to feminist critique of kenosis, 118
  on silent prayer, 115–18
Craigo-Snell, Shannon, on Rahner's theology, 54–57
Crawford, Matthew, 171n.25
Creamer, Deborah, on limitedness, 128
creatureliness, 166n.6

D

death
  control of, 2–3, 11–12, 19
  death awareness movement, xiii, 14
  denial of, xii, 16–17
  depersonalization of, 8–10
  and dispossession, 108
  fear of, 108
  isolation in, 12–14
  medicalization of, xiii, 8–12
  —responses to, 23
  as separation of soul and body, 53
  as taboo, 13–14
  tame vs wild, 7–8
  as universal, 53
"Death with dignity"
  and intolerance of dependence, 51–52
  Maynard's advocacy for, 138
  and personal identity, 36
  as slogan, 47
dementia, 11, 122
dependence, 30, 51–52, 59
Descartes, René, 30, 158n.38
dignity, 85–86, 162n.24
  and authenticity, 36
  and autonomy, 36

disability, 101, 109–11, 127–28, 131, 145–50
disability theory, 128, 162n.29
Duns Scotus, John, 158n.38

E
eschatology, 106–7, 125–26
Eucharist
 and flourishing, 128
 foretaste of the heavenly banquet, 125–26
 and identity, 126
 as kenotic practice, 125, 127
 and proclamation, 124
 symbolism of, 124
euthanasia (active), 23–25
euthanasia (passive). *See* withdrawal of life-sustaining treatment
extraordinary treatment, 45

F
feminist theology, critique of kenosis, 117

G
Gaudium et spes
 principle of totality, 48–49
Gawande, Atul, xiii
Giddens, Anthony
 ontological security, 16–17
 sequestration, 13
Gorer, Geoffrey
 "The Pornography of Death," 13
Gregory of Nyssa, 118
Gregory the Great, 127
Groningen Protocol, 25
Gustafson, James, 89

H
Hampson, Daphne, 117
Harlan, Susan, 177n.14
Hauerwas, Stanley, xviii
 anthropodicy, 99–100
 church as polis, 94–95
 community, 93–94
 eschewing universal ethics, 89
 essay form, 169n.3
 ethic of dispossession, 104–9, 149
 —and joy, 174n.73
 kenotic Christology, 104–6
 liberalism, 95–98, 171n.27
 martyrdom, 102–4
 medicine, 98–100
 moral description, 90–92
 quandary ethics, 90
 synthesis of Barthian and Roman Catholic thought, 88
 theological method, 88
 tragedy, 96–98, 108
 virtues, 93, 108
 —compassion as dangerous, 100–102, 173n.54
 —patience, 110–11
 —saints as exemplars, 173n.58
Heidegger, Martin
 being toward death, xi
 influence on Rahner, 54–55
Hippocratic oath, 45
Hobbes, Thomas, 97–98
Hockey, Jennifer, and zones of social abandonment, 14
Holy Spirit, 42, 110, 118, 123–25, 147, 165n.60
hospice, 27
 Christian roots of modern hospice, 128–29
 defined, 22–23

I

Ignatian spirituality, 119
Illich, Ivan, and specific diseconomy, 15
institutions
   deinstitutionalization, xvii, 15–18, 27
   medicine as, 99–100
   and personalism, 48
   role of, xv
   as scripts, xvii
   and social imaginary, 142
isolation, xiii, 8, 13–14
   suffering and, 98–100

J

Jesus's death
   and baptism, 119–24
   connected with nativity in iconography, 176n.1
   and Eucharist, 124–30
   and judgment, 69–77
   as model of dispossession, 108
   nature of, 41–42, 113–14
   and resurrection, 113–14
   as surrender, 57, 85–86, 106–8
   transformation of death, 42
Johns Hopkins Case, 47

K

Kant, Immanuel, 30
Kaufman, Sharon
   medically timed dying, 12
   on Medicare, 35
Kelsey, David, 115
Kierkegaard, Søren, and death as uncertain certainty, 1

L

L'Arche, 109–10, 175n.75
   Jean Vanier scandal, 175n.75

Lewis, Alan, 176n.7, 178n.42
Locke, John, 30, 97, 157n.31
Lord's Supper. *See* Eucharist
Luther, Martin, 33, 120, 169n.28, 174n.70
Lysaught, M. Therese, on sacramental practices, 114–15, 127, 129

M

martyrdom
   agency of the martyrs, 121
   baptism as symbol of, 121
   and Eucharist, 125
   as quotidian practice, 122
   spirituality of, 58–59, 104, 148
Maynard, Brittany, on the modern social imaginary, 137–43
McCormick, Richard, xvii, 46–52
McGill, Arthur C., on *bronze* people, xii
medical assistance in dying (MAID). *See* physician-assisted suicide
medicine
   alleviation of pain, 43–44
   care vs. cure, 100, 110
   education and epistemology, 10
   as good, 6
   and liberalism, 94–99
   specialization of, 13
   technology, 8–9
   as tragic profession, 96–97
modernity, 152n.6
Montaigne, Michel de, on authenticity, 31
mortification, 57, 126–27
Mumford, James
   the "newone," 179n.11
   package-deal ethics, 157n.20
Murdoch, Iris, 111, 119, 146

N

narrative
  and medical diagnosis, 8
  and moral imagination, 131
  and practices, 130–31
  and truthfulness, 88–96
Nuland, Sherwin, on cultural implications of medical technologies, 6–7

O

O'Donovan, Oliver, 101

P

palliative care, 22
personalism, 48–49
physician-assisted suicide (PAS), 23–28, 43–44, 50–52, 140
  and abuse, 156n.10
  and compassion, 102
  ethics of, 143–47
  and moral description, 92
  terminology, 152n.4
Pinckaers, Servais, xviii, 58–59
Plato, 29
practices, xix
  and agency, 130
  baptism, 119–24
  Eucharist, 124–30
  as formative, 114–15
  prayer, 115–19
  sacramental, 114–15
prayer, 115–19, 148–49
  apophatic prayer, 115–16
  decentering of the self, 115
  examen, 119
  as kenotic practice, 117–19
  Lord's prayer and dependence, 176n.7
proportionalism, 49–50

Q

quality of life, 47, 162n.24, 162n.29

R

Rahner, Karl, xviii
  death as natural, 52–53
  death as personal, 54–56
  death as surrender, 56–57
  fundamental option, 54
  on nature of freedom, 165n.59
Rawls, John, 97
reflexivity, xiv, 4–5, 15–20, 140
Reiser, Stanley, 9
Ridenour, Autumn Alcott, 85–86
Rousseau, Jean-Jacques, 97
rule of double effect, 45
running, 96

S

Sandel, Michael, 97–98
Saunders, Dame Cicely, on influence of Christian faith, 128–29
Schleiermacher, Friedrich, 166n.2
Singer, Peter, 173n.54
Sonderegger, Katherine, and the fundamental analysis of the creaturely, 62
Still Alice, 178n.32
suicide. *See* physician-assisted suicide
Sulmasy, Daniel, 24

T

Taylor, Charles
  modern identity, xvii, 28–38
  —affirmation of ordinary life, 33–34
  —inwardness, 29–31
  —nature as moral source, 31–33
  social imaginaries, 20, 29
  subjectivation, 17, 155n.59

terminal sedation, 44–45
Tessman, Lisa, 5–6
theological anthropology, xvi, 61, 63
   and limits, 78, 84, 89, 128, 166n.6
theology of the cross (*theologia crucis*),
   108, 169n.28, 174n.70
Tippetts, Kara, 140–43
Tolstoy, Leo, 154n.39
transhumanism, xiii

V
Vanstone, Canon W. H., on waiting,
   85–86
Velleman, David, 26

W
Ward, Graham, 118
Warnock, Baroness Mary, on the duty
   to die, 27

Weber, Max
   on Luther, 33
   on the Protestant work ethic, 34
Westphal, Merold, 115
Williams, Rowan, and baptismal
   identity, 120–22
withdrawal of life-sustaining
   treatment, 43, 47–49, 91,
   160n.9, 162n.29
witness, 58–59, 103–4, 111, 121,
   124, 148–50
Wittgenstein, Ludwig, 93, 170n.16
woodworking, 93–94
Wordsworth, William
   "The Prelude," 31–32

Y
Yoder, John Howard, 95, 174n.71
   and tainted legacies, 175n.75

Travis Pickell

is an assistant professor of theology and ethics at
George Fox University, where he also directs the Character
Virtue Initiative and the Cornerstone Core curriculum.